Osteoporosis

Dr Rebecca Fox-Spencer

Dr Pam Brown

Osteoporosis
First published – April 2006

Published by
CSF Medical Communications Ltd
1 Bankside, Lodge Road, Long Hanborough
Oxfordshire, OX29 8LJ, UK
T +44 (0)1993 885370 F +44 (0)1993 881868
enquiries@bestmedicine.com
www.bestmedicine.com

We are always interested in hearing from anyone
who has anything to add to our Simple Guides.
Please send your comments to *editor@csfmedical.com*.

Author Dr Rebecca Fox-Spencer
Managing Editor Dr Eleanor Bull
Medical Editor Dr Pam Brown
Science Editor Dr Scott Chambers
Production Editor Emma Catherall
Layout Jamie McCansh and Julie Smith
Operations Manager Julia Savory
Publisher Stephen I'Anson

ISBN-10: 1-905466-11-0
ISBN-13: 978-190546-611-5

Printed in Italy.

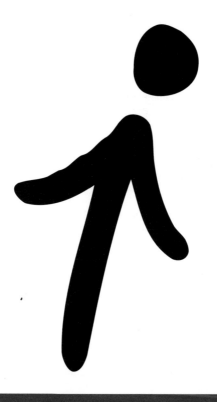

FOREWORD

TRISHA MACNAIR
Doctor and BBC Health Journalist

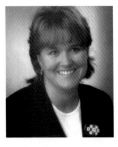 Getting involved in managing your own medical condition – or helping those you love or care for to manage theirs – is a vital step towards keeping as healthy as possible.

Whilst doctors, nurses and the rest of your healthcare team can help you with expert advice and guidance, nobody knows your body, your symptoms and what is right for *you* as well as you do.

There is no long-term (chronic) medical condition or illness that I can think of where the person concerned has absolutely no influence at all on their situation. The way you choose to live your life, from the food you eat to the exercise you take, will impact upon your disease, your well-being and how able you are to cope. You are in charge!

Being involved in making choices about your treatment helps you to feel in control of your problems, and makes sure you get the help that you really need. Research clearly shows that when people living with a chronic illness take an active role in looking after themselves, they can bring about significant improvements in their illness and vastly improve the quality of life they enjoy.

Of course, there may be occasions when you feel particularly unwell and it all seems out of your control. Yet most of the time there are plenty of things that you can do in order to reduce the negative effects that your condition can have on your life. This way you feel as good as possible and may even be able to alter the course of your condition.

So how do you gain the confidence and skills to take an active part in managing your condition, communicate with health professionals and work through sometimes worrying and emotive issues? The answer is to become better informed. Reading about your problem, talking to others who have been through similar experiences and hearing what the experts have to say will all help to build up your understanding and help you to take an active role in your own health care.

Simple Guides provide an invaluable source of help, giving you the facts that you need in order to understand the key issues and discuss them with your doctors and other professionals involved in your care. The information is presented in an accessible way but without neglecting the important details. Produced independently and under the guidance of medical experts *Osteoporosis* is an evidence-based, balanced and up-to-date review that I hope you will find enables you to play an active part in the successful management of your condition.

What happens normally?

WHAT HAPPENS NORMALLY?

We all appreciate that we couldn't possibly manage without our bones. But it is all too easy to assume that they are just lifeless 'scaffolding poles' and as long as they are there, they must be doing their job properly.

WHY DO WE NEED BONES?

Whilst some of the roles that your bones perform are obvious, there are others that you probably won't have been aware of. You can credit your bones with the ability to:

- support your body structure
- protect the organs inside your body (e.g. heart, lungs)
- provide anchoring points for internal parts of your body (e.g. muscles) to keep them in position
- act as a lever – working with your muscles to allow you to apply pushing and pulling forces
- store and produce blood cells
- store calcium and other minerals.

BONES ARE NOT ALL THE SAME

An adult skeleton contains 206 bones of a range of different shapes and sizes. Bone can be defined in terms of its:

- macroscopic structure (features which are visible to the naked eye)

- – long – a bone much longer than it is wide
- – short – a bone shaped almost like a cube, with a similar length and width
- – flat – a thin bone with a flat surface
- – irregular – bones of complex shape, with grooves or ridges, perhaps

- microscopic structure (features which are too small to be visible to the naked eye but can be seen under a microscope)
  - – compact (also known as *cortical* bone)
  - – spongy (also known as *trabecular* or *cancellous* bone).

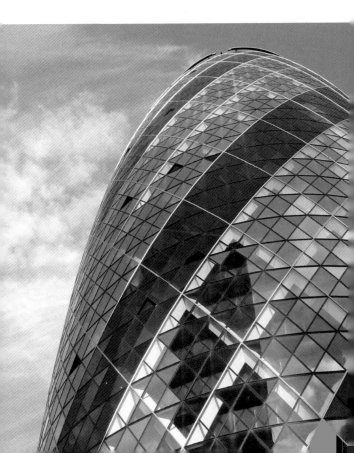

Generally, each bone is made up of spongy, trabecular tissue in the middle, with a compact layer of cortical bone surrounding and protecting it. The proportions of trabecular and cortical bone vary according to the bone's function. For example, long bones in the arms and legs which need a lot of strength have a lot of cortical bone compared with the irregular-shaped vertebrae in the spine.

Within the cavities inside long bones and in the spaces inside spongy, trabecular bone, is a substance called bone marrow. This can be either red or yellow, depending on the ratio of red blood cells to fat cells that it contains. One reason that bone marrow is important is because it is a source of **stem cells** – simple cells that differentiate into blood, fat, cartilage, nerve or bone cells. You will have probably heard a lot about stem cells in the news. The reason that they are of such great interest to medical researchers is because in the future it may be possible to use them to repair damaged tissue or grow completely new organs for people who need them.

Cells are the individual units that make up all the tissues in your body, like the brain, bone, heart and muscles. All living organisms are made up of at least one cell. The human body contains billions of them.

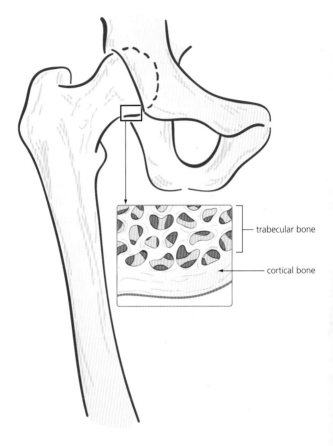

trabecular bone

cortical bone

THE ARRANGEMENT OF STRONG, CORTICAL BONE
AND SPONGY, TRABECULAR BONE IN THE HIP.

5

YOUR BONE IS ALIVE!

If you think that your bones are like lifeless scaffolding poles, you're wrong! Your bones are very much alive and continuously being regenerated. Bone tissue is broken down and replaced with new bone all the time – this is called bone turnover. The density of each of your bones varies naturally with age to a certain extent, and this happens because of a difference between the rate at which old bone is removed and the rate at which new bone is formed to replace it. Up until your early 30s, your bones are gradually becoming more dense, but beyond this point your bone starts to be broken down more quickly than it can be replaced, so your bone density falls. The density of your bones is one factor in determining their strength.

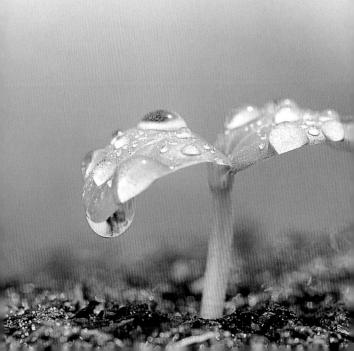

Bone resorption
(removal)

Bone formation

Gain bone
No change
Lose bone

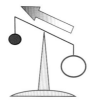

Up to the age of around 30

Formation of new bone
exceeds removal of old bone.
Bone density increases.

Gain bone
No change
Lose bone

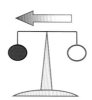

**Between the ages of about
30 and 35**

Removal of old bone is equal
to formation of new bone.
Bone density stays the same.

Gain bone
No change
Lose bone

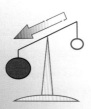

Over the age of 35

Removal of old bone exceeds
formation of new bone.
Bone density falls.

YOU CAN UNDERSTAND BONE TURNOVER
BY IMAGINING A SET OF SCALES.

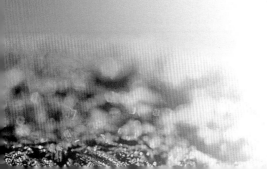

Although age is the most important factor determining which way the scales are tipped, there are other factors that influence the rate of bone removal and formation. Women who have gone through the menopause lose bone faster, as bone formation is maintained by the hormone oestrogen. When a woman reaches menopause, her oestrogen levels drop rapidly, and this causes a rapid phase of bone loss lasting 3 to 5 years, followed by continued slow bone loss long-term.

There are several other factors that affect how strong your bones are.

- **Genetics** – some ethnic groups (e.g. black people) have a tendency for stronger bones.

- **Diet** – certain components of your diet are crucial for strong healthy bones. We will look at this in more detail later.

- **Gender** – even before the menopause, women tend to have weaker bones than men of the same age.

- **Body weight** – heavier people tend to develop stronger bones to carry their extra weight.

- **Physical activity** – some types of regular weight-bearing and resistance exercise (working out with weights) increase the strength of the bones.

- **Hormones** – as well as the menopause, irregular periods in younger women can also be associated with bone loss. In men, low levels of testosterone can lead to weak bones.

- **Smoking and high alcohol intake** – both of these reduce bone density.

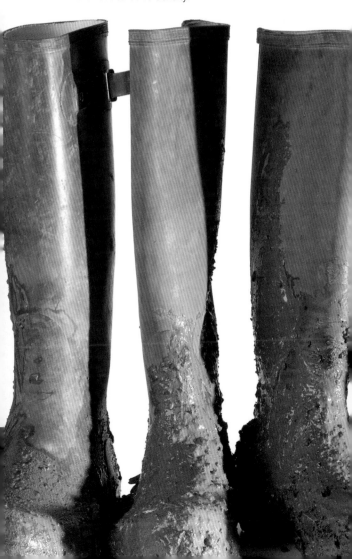

10

YOUR BONES HAVE NEEDS

It is important, particularly in childhood and adolescence whilst your bones are growing, that you give your bones everything they need to be as strong as possible. As well as partaking in regular exercise which puts weight on your bones and stimulates them to grow stronger, your bones need a number of nutrients from your diet.

- **Calcium** – the most abundant mineral in bone, is an essential component of its structure. We can get calcium from our diet. Foods like milk, other dairy products and oranges are rich in calcium.

- **Phosphate** – together with calcium, phosphate is a crucial component of the bone's structure. Phosphates can be found in most food types, in particular, eggs, milk, nuts and peas.

- **Vitamin D** – needed in order for your body to be able to absorb calcium from food. Most of the vitamin D you need is made in your skin on exposure to sunlight, but about 10% should also come from your diet.

The average adult skeleton contains 1 kg of calcium, which is the weight of a standard bag of sugar.

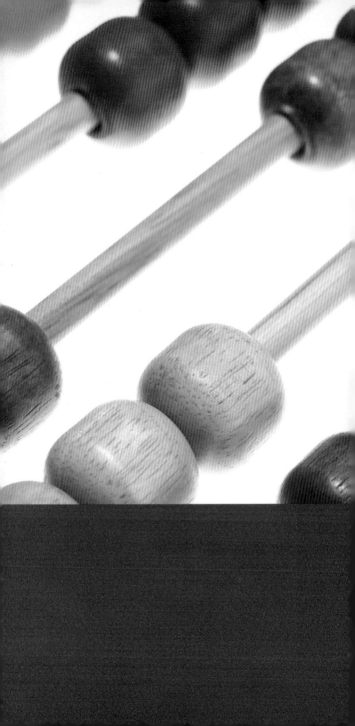

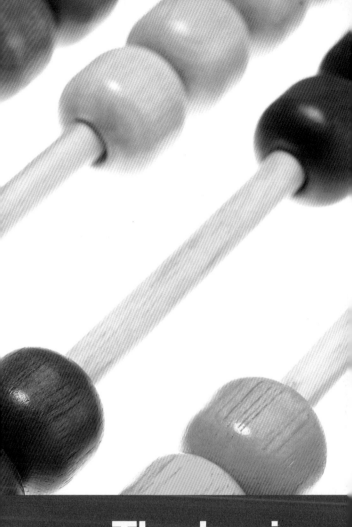

The basics

OSTEOPOROSIS – THE BASICS

If you have osteoporosis, your bones are
abnormally weak and liable to fracture. You will
need to adopt a 'bone-friendly' lifestyle and you
may need to take 'bone-preserving' drugs to stop
this risk increasing any further.

WHAT IS OSTEOPOROSIS?

The literal meaning of the word osteoporosis is
'holes in the bones', which is a pretty accurate
description of what happens if you have the
condition. In osteoporosis, the quality and the
density of bone tissue inside your bones
deteriorates, so that there is more empty space
inside them and therefore they become weaker.
This deterioration occurs in both cortical and
trabecular bone, so that both layers become thin
and weak. As a result of this deterioration, the
bone is more likely to break (fracture).

The main problem with having weak bones is
that they fracture more easily than they should.
This means that a minor fall, for example, which
would not normally cause a healthy bone to break,
can cause a painful and debilitating fracture. Even
a vigorous cough could result in a vertebral
fracture. Most people with osteoporosis only find
they have the disease when an X-ray reveals that
they have a fracture. If you have osteoporosis, the
bones most at risk of fracture are:
- wrist bones
- hip bones
- spinal bones (vertebrae).

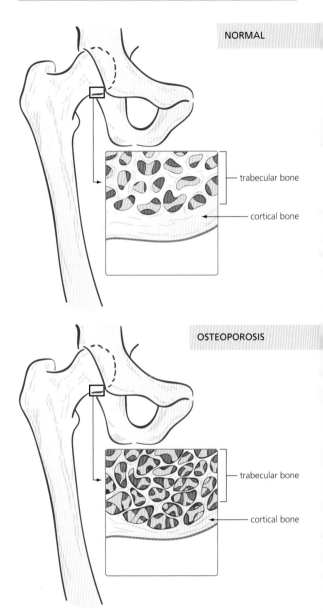

NORMAL

trabecular bone

cortical bone

OSTEOPOROSIS

trabecular bone

cortical bone

CHANGES TO THE STRUCTURE OF A HIP
BONE IN A PERSON WITH OSTEOPOROSIS.

WHY IS OSTEOPOROSIS A PROBLEM?

Aside from the obvious inconvenience of having a fracture, there are a number of ways in which fractures can impact on your life:

- being less mobile

- losing your independence

- feeling isolated

- worry over the risk of further fractures

- loss of height and development of a stooped back (because of fractures in the vertebrae of the spine)

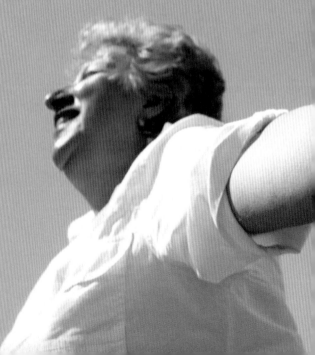

an increased risk of premature death,
particularly after a hip or spine fracture, due to
infections or extended bed rest causing blood
clots or pneumonia.

When a bone breaks as a result of a trivial trauma,
such as coughing, falling from a standing position,
bending or reaching, it is called a 'fragility fracture'.

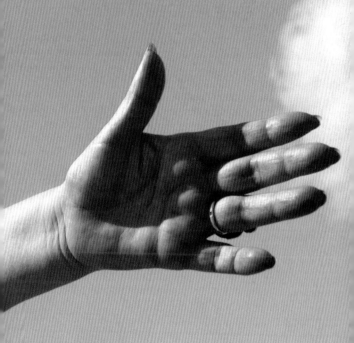

IF IT IS WELL MANAGED, THERE IS NO REASON WHY HAVING
OSTEOPOROSIS SHOULD RESTRICT YOUR INDEPENDENCE.

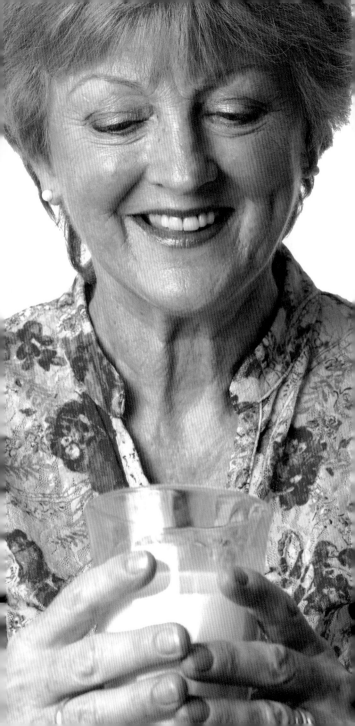

WHAT CAUSES OSTEOPOROSIS?

As we saw earlier, there are many factors that affect how strong your bones are. Anything which reduces your bone strength will contribute to you developing osteoporosis.

- **Increasing age** – beyond the age of about 35, bone density decreases. Osteoporosis mainly affects men and women over the age of 50.

- **Menopause** – when oestrogen levels fall after the menopause, bone density decreases too. Postmenopausal women represent the largest group of people with osteoporosis.

- **Low testosterone** – in men, the hormone testosterone slows bone resorption in a similar manner to oestrogen in women. Low testosterone levels in men can cause reduced bone density and can lead to osteoporosis.

- **Genetic tendencies** – your family history and your ethnicity can increase your risk of developing osteoporosis. People of Caucasian or Asian origin are statistically more at risk of developing osteoporosis.

- **Other diseases** – some diseases can affect normal bone turnover and therefore increase the risk of osteoporosis (e.g. kidney failure, liver disease).

■ **Drugs** – some drugs used to treat other conditions can also affect bone turnover and therefore cause osteoporosis (e.g. steroids and thyroid hormones).

■ **Low body weight** – very petite people are at particular risk of osteoporosis.

■ **Poor diet** – a lack of foods rich in calcium or vitamin D (such as milk, cheese, oily fish) in the diet can contribute to osteoporosis.

■ **Smoking/excessive alcohol consumption** – both of these factors reduce the strength of bone and can potentially lead to osteoporosis.

■ **Lack of exercise** – bones need to be stressed by having weight put through them, particularly whilst they are growing, in order to gain strength. An inactive lifestyle increases the chances that you will get osteoporosis

■ **Pregnancy and breast-feeding** – rarely, a woman might develop osteoporosis during pregnancy, though the reasons for this are unclear. Usually the bones recover after the woman has stopped breast-feeding.

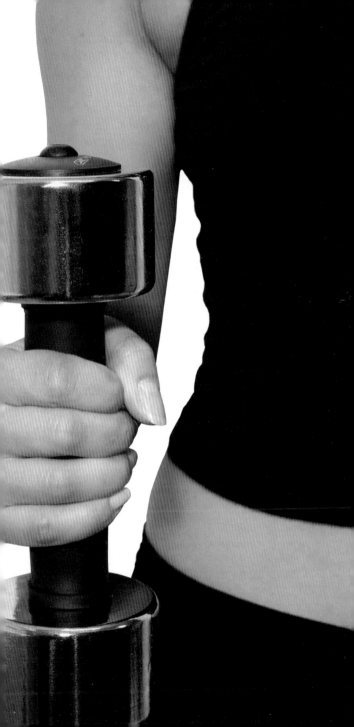

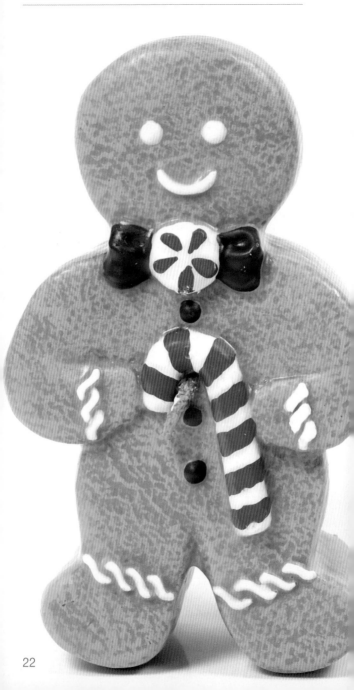

HOW DO YOU KNOW IF YOU HAVE OSTEOPOROSIS?

One of the major difficulties when it comes to managing osteoporosis is knowing that it's happening in the first place! It is often nicknamed 'the silent disease', because it doesn't cause any obvious symptoms until the first fracture occurs. As we will see later, osteoporosis can be suspected or diagnosed on the basis of specific scans that are done in hospital, but it is unlikely that you will have one of these unless you have already had a fracture, or are at a very clearly increased risk of osteoporosis (due to your age, a family history of osteoporosis, and long-term treatment with steroids, for example).

Most often then, a fracture is the first indication of osteoporosis. Even this can be easy to miss though! Some people (and their doctors) wrongly assume that the discomfort that is being caused by vertebral fractures is just everyday back pain. Repeated vertebral (spinal) fractures often cause a loss of height and a stooped back. Hip and wrist fractures are usually obvious and need expert hospital management.

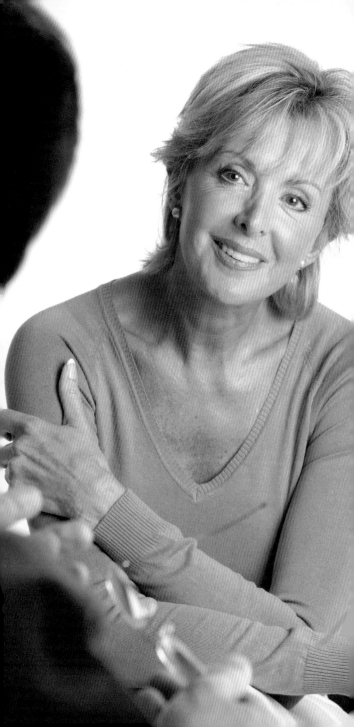

WHEN SHOULD YOU GO TO THE DOCTOR?

Don't be afraid to visit your doctor and ask for their advice if you are at all concerned that you may be at risk of osteoporosis. In particular, you should go and see your doctor if:

- you have previously had a fracture

- you suffer severe, incapacitating back pain

- you are postmenopausal and your mother or father had a hip fracture before the age of 75.

Osteoporosis and osteoarthritis

Some people get a little confused as to the difference between osteoporosis and osteoarthritis. Osteoporosis affects the strength of the bones, whereas osteoarthritis is specifically a problem with the joints between them. Osteoarthritis occurs when the cartilage and lubricating fluid which cushion bones at the joints start to disappear. This can result in bones rubbing against each other when joints move, affecting the range of movement and causing joint stiffness and pain. It can also cause backache, due to rubbing together of the vertebrae, and this symptom can be confused with the back pain caused by osteoporosis. Osteoporosis, however, doesn't cause any symptoms until the first fracture occurs.

For more information see
Arthritis

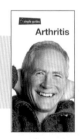

DIAGNOSING OSTEOPOROSIS

If you go to your doctor with concerns you may
have about osteoporosis they will want to know
about any previous fractures and whether there is
a history of osteoporosis in your family. He or she
will also consider any other medical conditions you
have, or treatments you are taking, in case they
are increasing your risk of osteoporosis.

If your doctor suspects that you might have
osteoporosis, the only definitive way for this to be
diagnosed is by a type of scan called a DXA (dual
X-ray absorptiometry) scan. DXA directly measures
bone density at the hip and spine, and will usually
be carried out in a hospital.

Your measured bone density will then be
compared with the average measurements for a
healthy young adult of your gender to provide a
'T-score' for each site. We will look at T-scores in
more detail later on (see *Managing osteoporosis*
page 78). Your doctor may decide, on the basis of
your symptoms and history, to start treating you
for osteoporosis before you have had the scan,
particularly if there is a long waiting list.

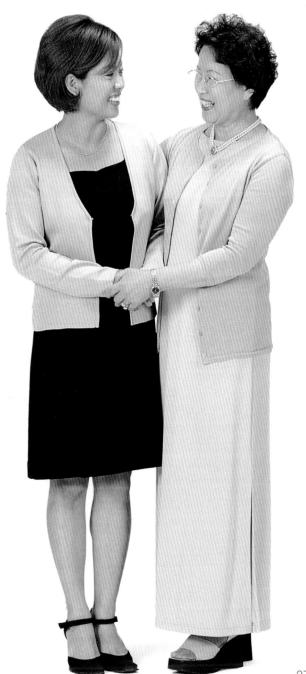

MANAGING OSTEOPOROSIS

If you are diagnosed with osteoporosis, there are various approaches that you and your doctor can take to ensure that it is managed as effectively as possible. If you are at risk of osteoporosis, but your bone density has not fallen low enough for it to be considered osteoporosis, there are plenty of steps you can take to minimise the risk that you will develop it in the future.

Lifestyle changes

Whether you are at risk of developing osteoporosis or already have it, it is always a good idea to:

■ ensure you eat a balanced diet with plenty of calcium

■ ask your doctor whether you can take vigorous weight-bearing exercise (e.g. aerobics or jogging) or resistance exercise (working out with weights)

■ if you smoke, try to quit

■ reduce your alcohol intake

■ try to expose your hands, forearms and face to sunlight for 15–20 minutes per day during the summer months.

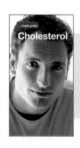

For more information see
Cholesterol

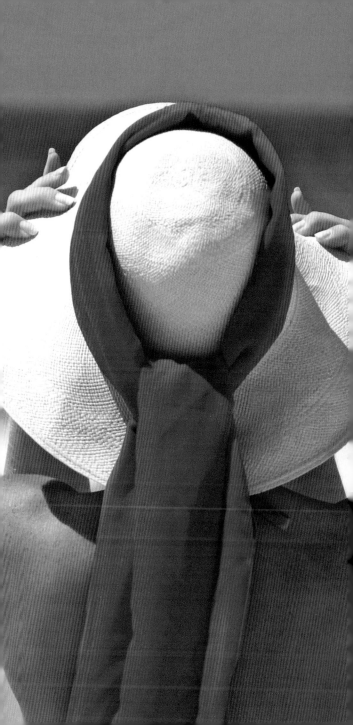

Prevention of fractures

Given that the main problem with osteoporosis is the increased risk of fractures, you should try to minimise the risk of these in your own home. We will look at this in more detail in *Managing osteoporosis* (see page 118), but in general:

- minimise clutter on your floors and always wear sensible shoes

- mop up spillages immediately and seal down corners of rugs/carpets

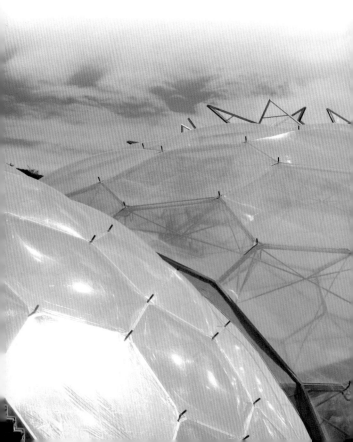

- ensure good visibility – turn on lights if it is dark and have your sight tested regularly

- fit non-slip mats and grab/hand rails

- ask your doctor whether any of your current medications may be affecting your balance (such as those to control your blood pressure and heart rate, for example). Also ask about high dose calcium and vitamin D supplements that may help to reduce 'body sway' and muscle weakness and make other bone-sparing treatments work better.

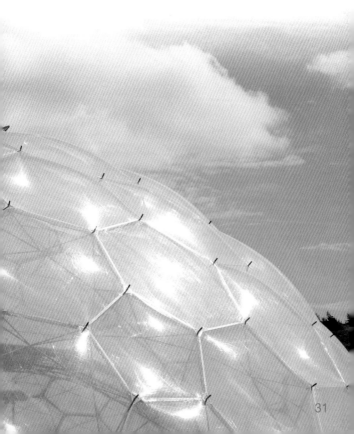

Drug treatments

There is a growing range of drugs available to your doctor for treating osteoporosis:

- bisphosphonates (e.g. alendronic acid [Fosamax®], risedronate sodium [Actonel®])
- dual action bone agents (strontium ranelate [Protelos®])
- selective oestrogen receptor modulators (abbreviated to SERMs; e.g. raloxifene hydrochloride [Evista®])
- parathyroid hormone (e.g. teriparatide [Forsteo®])
- calcitriol (Rocaltrol®, Calcijex®)
- calcitonin (Miacalcic®)
- hormone replacement therapy.

All of the different management strategies are covered in more detail in the *Managing osteoporosis* section.

Pain management

If you are suffering from long-term pain because of osteoporosis, the doctor may suggest that you try some pain management strategies. These could include:

- 'analgesic' (pain-killing) drugs, by mouth, injection or in patch form (e.g. aspirin, morphine)
- physiotherapy, including exercises in water (hydrotherapy)
- transcutaneous electrical nerve stimulation (TENS, interrupts the pain signals travelling to your brain by means of electrode pads attached to the skin)
- relaxation training
- complementary therapies (including acupuncture).

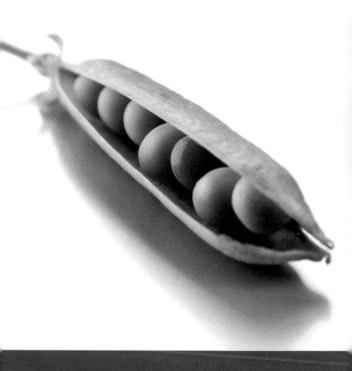

Why me?

WHY ME?

If you have osteoporosis, or are caring for someone with the condition, you are certainly not alone. It is the most common bone disease known to man and is estimated to affect more than 100 million people worldwide.

HOW COMMON IS OSTEOPOROSIS?

In order to assess how many people have osteoporosis, we have to look at the number of people suffering fractures. The most recent estimate is that half of women and one-fifth of men over the age of 50 in the UK will suffer a fracture (that's over 5 million women and nearly 2 million men, *National Osteoporosis Society*). Although we cannot be certain about the exact proportion, many of these fractures will be due to osteoporosis, and many will also go untreated. Osteoporosis is more common in western countries such as the UK than in some developing countries. This is somewhat surprising, given that people in more developed regions tend to have a lot more calcium in their diets. However, other factors such as longer life-expectancy, lack of exercise, excessive drinking of alcohol and smoking probably contribute to the increased risk of osteoporosis in the UK compared with poorer areas of the world.

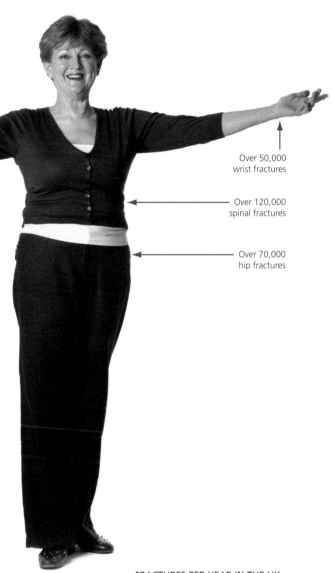

Over 50,000
wrist fractures

Over 120,000
spinal fractures

Over 70,000
hip fractures

FRACTURES PER YEAR IN THE UK.
Source: National Osteoporosis Society, www.nos.org.uk

WHY DO I HAVE OSTEOPOROSIS?

At any age, the overall risk of osteoporosis depends on:

- the peak bone density achieved in the teenage years
- the age at which bone loss begins
- the rate at which bone loss progresses.

You are at increased risk of developing osteoporosis if you:

- are female
- are a postmenopausal woman (particularly if the menopause started before you were 45)
- are a woman who has had a hysterectomy before the age of 45
- are elderly – your risk increases with age
- are of Caucasian or Asian ethnicity
- are petite in build
- have irregular periods
- are inactive for long periods of time (e.g. due to bed rest following an operation)
- have too little calcium in your diet
- smoke or drink too much alcohol
- have a history of osteoporosis in your family.

Whilst doctors know that these factors will increase your risk of osteoporosis, many cases of the disease are described as idiopathic. This means that the specific cause of osteoporosis is unknown.

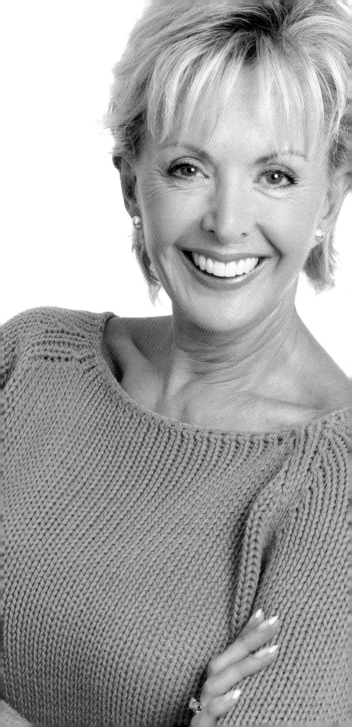

CALCULATE YOUR OWN BODY MASS INDEX (BMI)

It's very simple to work out your own BMI, to see whether your weight has put you at risk of osteoporosis. Grab a tape measure, a set of bathroom scales and a calculator and follow these two steps.

■ Measure your height in metres. Multiply this number by itself and write down the answer, for example:

$$1.80 \text{ (metres)} \times 1.80 = 3.24$$

■ Measure your weight in kilograms. Divide it by the number you wrote down in the first step, for example:

$$80 \text{ (kilograms)} \div 3.24 = 24.7$$

The number you get is your BMI. As a general rule, for adults aged over 20, the BMI relates to the following:

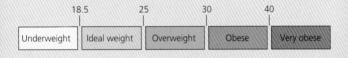

	18.5	25	30	40	
Underweight	Ideal weight	Overweight	Obese	Very obese

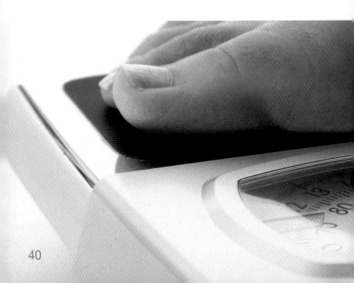

Secondary osteoporosis

When bone strength is reduced by another medical problem or its treatment, this is sometimes referred to as secondary osteoporosis. A number of medications can cause osteoporosis, such as steroids (used for asthma, for example) and immunosuppressants (used after organ transplants and during cancer treatment). The health problems that can cause low bone density include the following.

■ **Hypogonadism** – although this can refer to low oestrogen levels in women, more commonly it describes abnormally low levels of testosterone in men, affecting approximately one in every two hundred men in the UK. Oestrogen and testosterone both act in the body to sustain bone density.

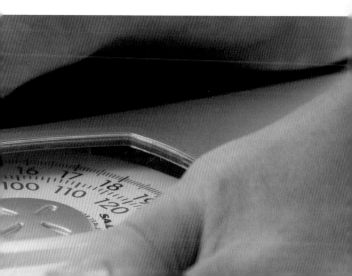

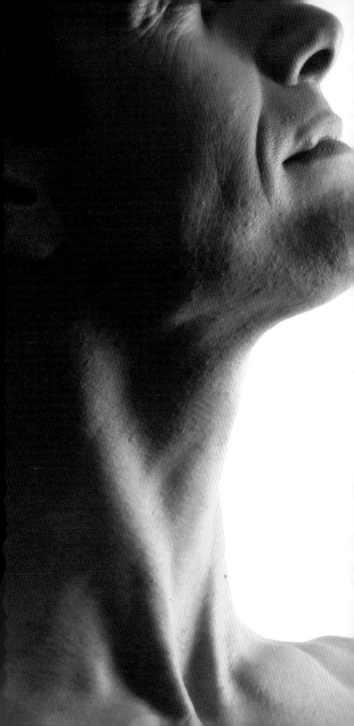

- **Hyperparathyroidism** – abnormally high levels of parathyroid hormone (which helps regulate the concentration of calcium in the blood), affects around one in every thousand people. Although daily injections of this hormone can be used to treat osteoporosis, persistently high levels can increase the rate of bone removal.

- **Hyperthyroidism** – abnormally high levels of thyroid hormone (produced in the body or as a result of over-replacement with thyroxine tablets), affects about 1% of women but only one in every thousand men in the UK. Excess thyroid hormone increases the rate of bone removal.

- **Cushing's syndrome** – a rare condition (only around 5 new cases per million people each year) where the body is exposed to high levels of the hormone cortisol, causing symptoms such as obesity, fragile skin, weakness, anxiety and depression. Cortisol is a naturally-occurring steroid, and Cushing's syndrome can cause osteoporosis in the same way as long-term treatment with steroid drugs.

- **Rheumatoid arthritis** – a long-term condition which can be very painful, characterised by inflammation in the linings of the joints between the bones. It affects around one in every hundred people, usually between the ages of 30 and 50. Having arthritis can limit your level of activity, which can contribute to developing osteoporosis.

- **Cystic fibrosis** – an inherited disease that affects organs such as the lungs, filling them with sticky mucus and stopping them from working properly. It currently affects around 7,500 people in the UK. There is an increased risk of osteoporosis due to direct effects on bone turnover, hypogonadism, problems with absorbing nutrients from food, poor mobility and the use of steroid drugs.

- **Inflammatory bowel disease** – a condition where the intestine gets red and swollen, affecting the way your body absorbs nutrients such as calcium and vitamin D from your diet.

- **Coeliac disease** – caused by an inability to digest gluten (a protein found in wheat), this disease prevents you from being able to absorb nutrients such as calcium and vitamin D properly.

- **Eating disorders** – e.g. anorexia and bulimia, again limit the amount of calcium and vitamin D available for bone strengthening.

- **Gastrointestinal problems** – can affect the absorption of nutrients from food.

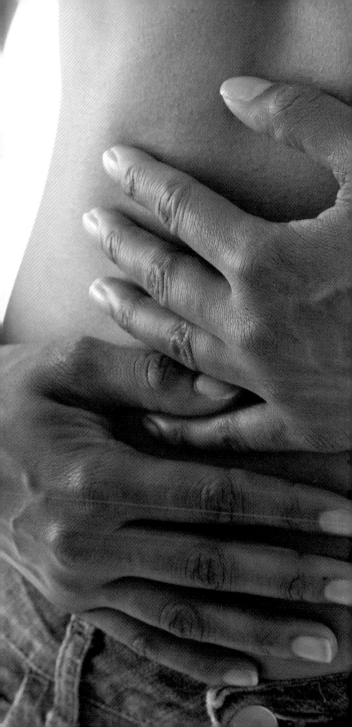

■ **Kidney disease** – problems with the kidneys affect the way that the body controls the levels of nutrients such as calcium and phosphate. This can lead to loss of bone strength.

■ **Liver disease** – the liver is responsible for making new substances in the body, converting substances of one type to another, and controlling how energy is distributed. Unsurprisingly, if the liver is not working properly, this affects all sorts of processes in the body, including the maintenance of healthy bones.

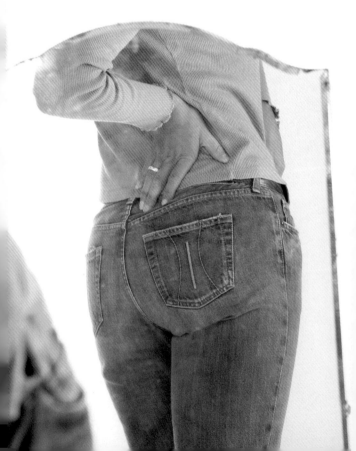

- **Severe chronic obstructive pulmonary disease (COPD)** – a long-term and incurable lung condition that often affects people who smoke.

- **Injury to the spinal cord** – reduces bone density mainly due to the lack of weight-bearing exercise.

THE FEMALE ATHLETE TRIAD

The female athlete triad refers to three related health issues:

- eating disorders
- absence of periods (amenorrhoea)
- osteoporosis.

This triad of problems is particularly common amongst female athletes, as the name suggests, but can also affect any woman who is excessively concerned with their weight and body shape.

These three problems can occur when a woman uses potentially harmful, and often ineffective, methods to achieve their 'ideal' shape and weight. Excessive exercise and eating disorders can reduce a woman's oestrogen levels, causing problems with the menstrual cycle, as demonstrated by the amenorrhoea, and increasing the risk of osteoporosis in later life. We will look at the role of oestrogen in osteoporosis in more detail in *Simple science* page 62.

Remember that the way you treat your body now can have a critical bearing on your future health.

HOW WILL OSTEOPOROSIS AFFECT ME?

Having a low bone density will not affect the quality of life you enjoy. It is the fractures that can result from a low bone density that will impact upon the way you live and may stop you from doing certain things. Vertebral (spine) fractures in particular are not always painful and so they may go unnoticed. However, a number of vertebral fractures over time can cause you to develop a stooped back (sometimes known as dowager's hump) and to lose height.

Fractures to the wrists or elsewhere in the arms or legs are more easily identifiable and can be quite debilitating because the affected limb will be out of action for some time. Hip fracture, however, is the most problematic.

Hip fracture requires surgical repair, a period of hospitalisation and rehabilitation, and most people do not regain their pre-fracture mobility and independence. Alongside the immediate pain that may accompany a fracture when it occurs, there will often be long-term, 'chronic' pain and restricted mobility following a fracture, particularly with multiple vertebral fractures. Often, this will lead to the need for help in the home from a relative, friend or carer, and therefore some loss of independence.

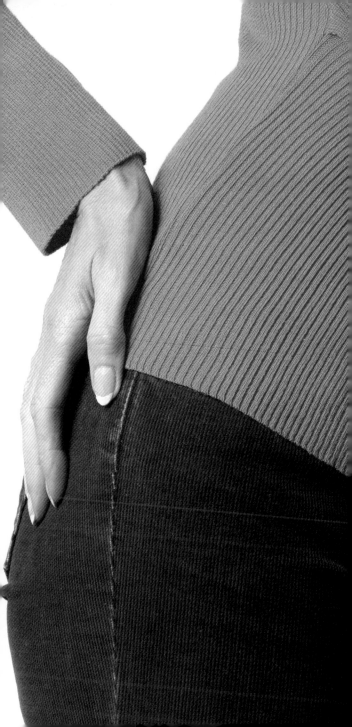

Clearly, avoiding fractures is crucial if you want to minimise the impact that osteoporosis can have on your life. This is why it is so important to get an early diagnosis from your doctor and to start treatment to slow down the rate at which you lose bone. A combination of drug treatment, improvements to your diet and exercise levels and taking measures to reduce the risk of falls in your home are generally effective in minimising the risk of future fractures.

OSTEOPOROSIS IN MEN

Osteoporosis has a reputation of being a female problem, as men generally have denser bones than women. Although it is indeed true that the majority of people who have the condition are postmenopausal women, significant numbers of men over the age of 50 suffer fractures, and many of these are due to osteoporosis. Although there are many cases of idiopathic osteoporosis in men, the majority of cases are secondary to some other cause, such as low levels of testosterone (hypogonadism) or long-term use of steroid drugs for conditions like asthma. Men tend to smoke more and drink more alcohol than women too. If you are a man, it is very easy to dismiss osteoporosis as something that will not happen to you, but the figures speak for themselves. You need to look after your bones too!

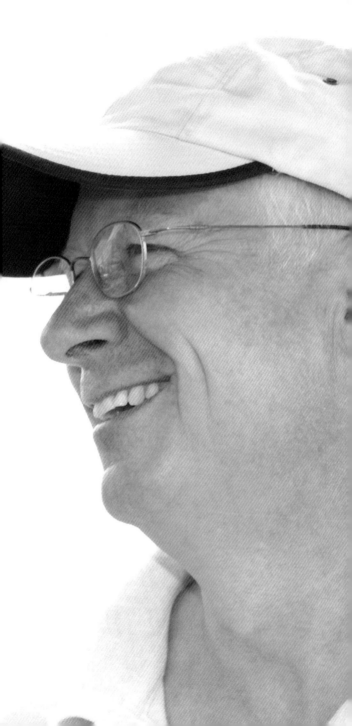

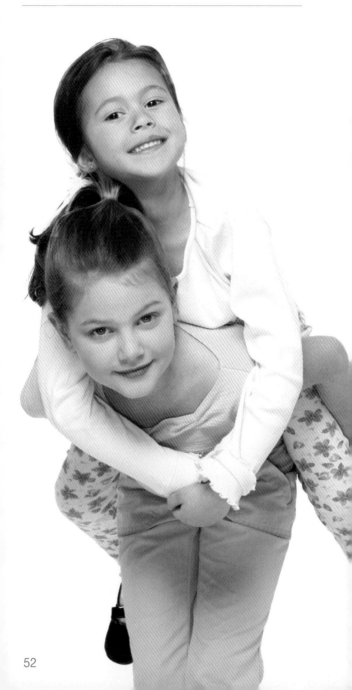

OSTEOPOROSIS IN CHILDREN

Children are certainly not at high risk of osteoporosis, but this does not mean that bone health should be ignored during childhood, since this time is critical in achieving peak bone density. It is vital that your child's bones are given everything they need to grow and gain strength at this crucial stage. Rarely, osteoporosis can occur in children, most often due to specific medical conditions or the long-term use of medications, as we have already seen. In some cases, there may be no identifiable cause, and a child will be diagnosed with idiopathic juvenile osteoporosis. At present, however, this is thought to affect fewer than 100 children in the UK.

The symptoms of osteoporosis in children are similar to those in adults, including:

- fractures

- pain in the back, legs, hips and feet

- difficulty in walking

- stooping and/or lower than average height.

There is a condition similar to osteoporosis which may occur during childhood. Osteogenesis imperfecta (commonly known as brittle bone disease) is caused by a lack of collagen, a protein which provides strength inside your bones. It is different from osteoporosis which, as you know, develops over time and is caused by an overall loss of bone, rather than the specific lack of collagen protein. However, like osteoporosis, osteogenesis imperfecta causes an increased risk of fractures.

OSTEOPOROSIS DURING PREGNANCY

As we have seen, osteoporosis is most likely to
affect women once they reach menopause and so it
is not a major health issue during pregnancy.
However, particularly when there is a history of
eating disorders or coeliac disease (the condition
caused by an inability to digest gluten), for example,
pregnancy can apparently bring on osteoporosis.

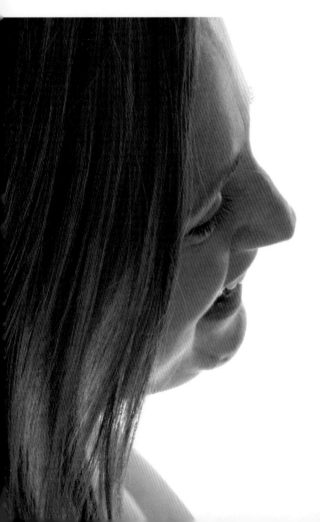

Pregnancy-associated osteoporosis usually occurs during the last stage of pregnancy (weeks 28–40) or shortly after the birth. It is generally a temporary condition and mainly occurs in a mother's first pregnancy. Breast-feeding can also cause a temporary reduction in bone density, but this tends to resolve once breast-feeding has ceased.

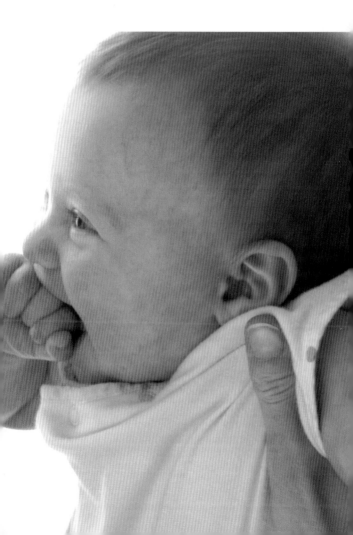

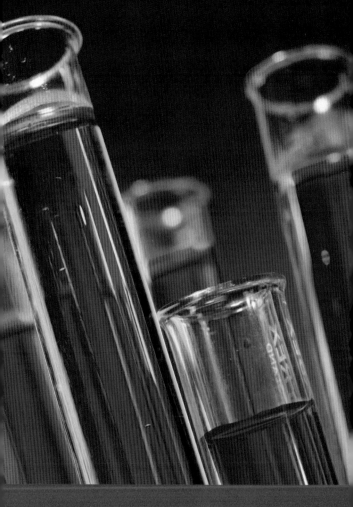

Simple
science

SIMPLE SCIENCE

In order to understand how the various treatments for osteoporosis work, it will be useful to learn a little more about exactly what is going wrong in your bones when you have the disease.

BONE TURNOVER

As we saw in the *What happens normally?* section, your bone is constantly being renewed – old bone tissue is broken down and new bone is formed to replace it. Together, these events are known as bone remodelling or turnover, and are due to the actions of two distinct types of cell in the bone.

- **Osteoclasts** break down bone using acids and enzymes (a process technically known as bone resorption). An enzyme is a protein that speeds up chemical reactions.

- **Osteoblasts** create new bone to replace that removed by the osteoclasts (bone formation).

Once you reach the age of 35, your bone density starts to fall as the rate of bone resorption exceeds the rate of bone formation. Clearly then, as you get older, your bone density will naturally drop below that which you had as a healthy young adult. However, if this difference becomes larger (that is, your bone density drops lower), you are defined as having osteopenia or low bone density. If the difference becomes larger still, you have osteoporosis.

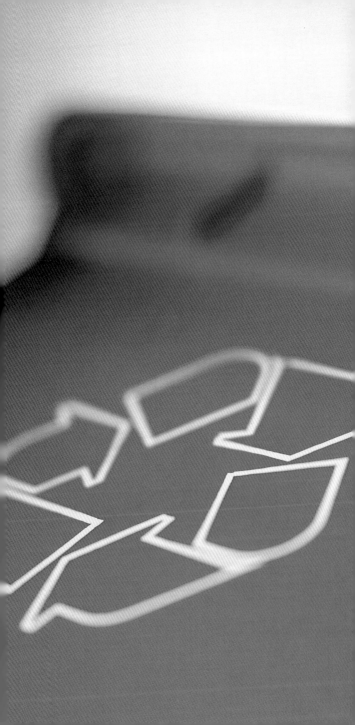

Remember the scales analogy we used earlier? One way to treat osteoporosis is to try and balance the scales, either by reducing the rate of bone resorption and/or increasing the rate at which new bone is made. The drugs available for treating osteoporosis work by directly affecting the rate of bone turnover.

Bone resorption ● (removal)   Bone formation ○

■ **Bisphosphonates** reduce the rate of bone resorption.

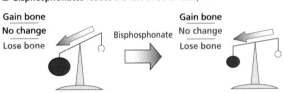

■ **Parathyroid hormone (teriparatide)** increases the rate of new bone formation.

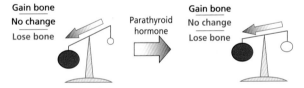

■ **Strontium ranelate** decreases the rate of bone resorption **and** increases the rate of new bone formation.

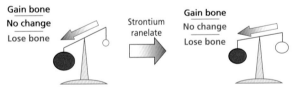

DRUGS FOR OSTEOPOROSIS ACT TO RESTORE THE BALANCE OF BONE FORMATION AND RESORPTION.

BONE STRUCTURE

We have already seen that calcium and to a certain extent, phosphate, are important components of your diet when it comes to maintaining healthy bones. The reason for this becomes clear when you look in more detail at what bone is made of. Both compact, cortical bone and spongy, trabecular bone contain a matrix, which is almost entirely composed of collagen fibres. These are white, non-stretchy fibres with lots of tensile strength (in other words, strong when you **PULL** against them). However, in order for your bones to have compressional strength as well (in other words, strong when you **PUSH** against them), this matrix must be fortified by deposits of bone salts. This is where the calcium and phosphate come in – they are both essential components of the major bone salt (known as hydroxyapatite).

Most foods contain sufficient amounts of phosphate and it is, therefore, more common for a lack of calcium or vitamin D to compromise bone strength than a lack of phosphate. As we saw in the *What happens normally?* section, vitamin D is needed for the body to be able to absorb calcium from food in the gut. Most of your vitamin D is made in your skin on exposure to sunlight, but you still need to supplement this with vitamin D from your diet.

The bone matrix is largely composed of collagen fibres and hydroxyapatite, a bone salt that is made up of calcium and phosphate.

HORMONES AND BONE STRENGTH

Oestrogen

The most important cause of osteoporosis is the reduction in oestrogen levels which occurs in women at menopause. A woman's ovaries start making oestrogen at puberty, and this hormone helps limit the amount of bone resorption all the way through to the menopause. This is because oestrogen reduces the activity of the osteoclast cells which carry out bone resorption, and some experts believe that the hormone may even kill these cells off. Therefore, at the menopause when oestrogen levels fall, the rate of bone resorption will start to rise, thereby causing bone to be lost more quickly.

Any event which reduces the overall time that a woman produces oestrogen, such as an early menopause or removal of the ovaries, can increase the risk of osteoporosis later in life.

A hormone is a naturally occurring substance, made by specialised cells in the body. It travels in the bloodstream and affects the activity of cells elsewhere in the body.

A DROP IN OESTROGEN LEVELS
CAN IMPAIR BONE STRENGTH.

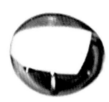

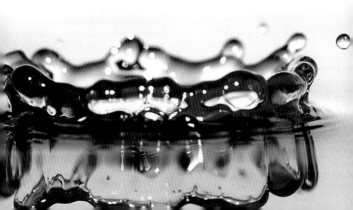

In the past, hormone replacement therapy (HRT) has been used as a treatment for osteoporosis. This is because HRT restores the levels of oestrogen to what they were before the menopause, thus preventing the rate of bone resorption from getting too high. However, there is some evidence that the effects of supplementary oestrogen in HRT leads to an increase in the risk of breast cancer and problems with the heart and blood vessels, for example. HRT is therefore no longer recommended as a treatment for osteoporosis.

More recently, a class of drugs called the selective oestrogen receptor modulators (or SERMs) has been developed. A receptor is a tiny structure which responds to a specific substance by causing some effect in the body, and oestrogen exerts all of its effects by attaching to oestrogen receptors. The SERMs, however, are able to bind to these same receptors. They are known as selective because in some regions of the body (such as in the breast), they prevent oestrogen from acting, but in other regions (such as the bone), SERMs mimic the action of oestrogen when they bind to the receptors. Due to the fact that SERMs reduce the effects of oestrogen at the breast, SERMs do not carry the same risk of breast cancer as HRT. Their specific effect on bone, however, makes SERMs effective drugs for treating osteoporosis and the spine but not the hip.

For more information on SERMs (e.g. raloxifene hydrochloride [Evista®]) refer to the *Managing osteoporosis* (page 104) section or speak to your GP.

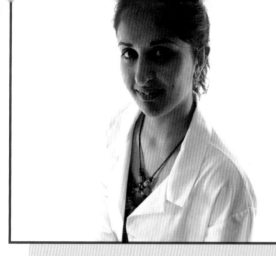

PHARMACIST

As a pharmacist I offer you essential services like drug dispensing and self-care support, within your local area. I can also provide you with lifestyle advice (such as what to include in a healthy diet).

Pharmacists within the community now play a much bigger role than ever before in helping people to manage their long-term conditions. This may involve keeping track of which medications you are using and how often you are taking them.

A number of new schemes have been laid out in our new pharmacy contract, which reflects the government's health priorities: support for self-care, management of long-term conditions and public health. By increasing the range of services that we can offer, we can improve the level of care and support that you, as a patient with a long-term condition like osteoporosis, can expect from your health service.

Testosterone

As we have already seen, osteoporosis can affect men as well as women, and hormone levels can play a part in men too. Men have some oestrogen, though much less than women. More important in men is the role of the male hormone, testosterone, which is made in the testicles. If the amount of testosterone produced is abnormally low, the man is described as having hypogonadism. This is one of the major causes of osteoporosis in men. There are a number of reasons that too little testosterone might be made.

- You can inherit problems that reduce your testosterone production, such as Klinefelter's syndrome, in which the testicles do not grow properly and so produce very little of the hormone.

- Inflammation or injury of the testicles can impair testosterone production.

- Alcohol reduces testosterone levels, so excessive alcohol consumption can increase the risk of osteoporosis.

- Middle-aged and older men naturally produce less testosterone than younger men.

- Radiation or chemotherapy, used to treat cancer, are both thought to reduce testosterone levels. Also, if you have prostate cancer, your doctor may try to reduce your testosterone levels with medication or surgery, as some prostate tumours are 'fuelled' by the hormone.

Some cases of hypogonadism can be managed by removing the cause, such as treating inflammation of the testicles or drinking less alcohol. However, in some cases, the best option is to take testosterone supplements.

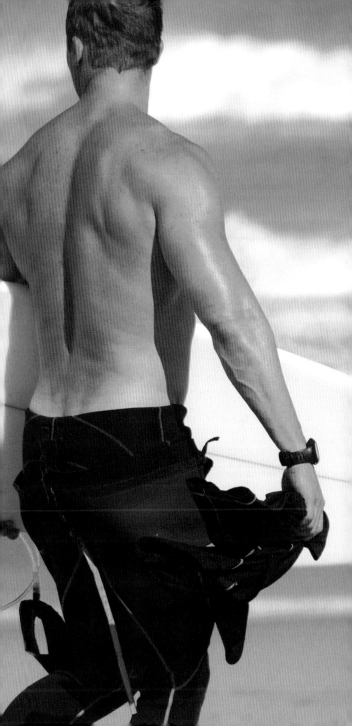

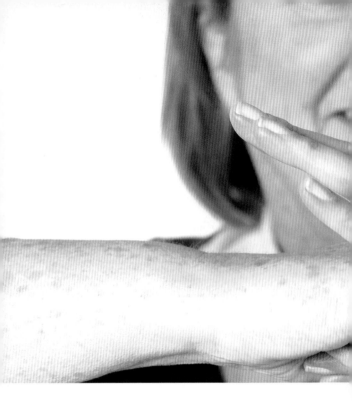

Parathyroid hormone

Aside from oestrogen and testosterone, another hormone plays an important role in regulating bone strength. Parathyroid hormone, produced in the parathyroid glands in the neck, controls the movement of calcium and phosphate between the bones and the blood. Calcium and phosphate are required for compressional strength in bone (as we saw earlier), so parathyroid hormone can affect bone strength by increasing or decreasing levels of these nutrients inside the bones. If levels of vitamin D fall, this triggers an increase in the level of parathyroid hormone. This allows blood calcium levels to be maintained, though this is at the expense of calcium leaching out of the bones.

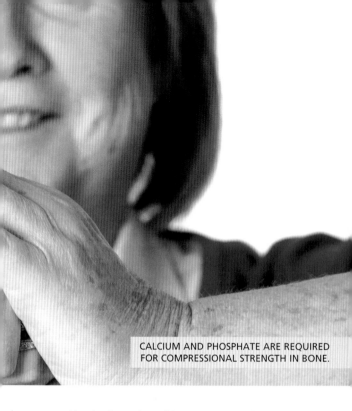

CALCIUM AND PHOSPHATE ARE REQUIRED FOR COMPRESSIONAL STRENGTH IN BONE.

If levels of parathyroid hormone are too high (caused by hyperparathyroidism, in which the parathyroid glands are overactive, or there is too little vitamin D, also causing excessive levels of parathyroid hormone), this can lead to bone loss.

On the other hand small amounts of parathyroid hormone given daily to a person with osteoporosis can stimulate bone formation. As a result, parathyroid hormone can be used as a treatment for osteoporosis, see *Managing osteoporosis* (page 106).

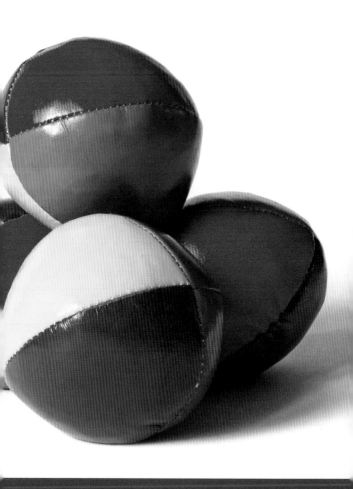

Managing osteoporosis

MANAGING OSTEOPOROSIS

By working in partnership with your doctor, you will be able to develop a strategy which keeps your osteoporosis under control, reduces the chance of future fractures and minimises the impact that these have on your life.

CATCHING IT EARLY

The first stage in managing osteoporosis properly is getting an accurate diagnosis from your doctor. Given that osteoporosis can be 'silent', in other words not showing any symptoms until the first fracture occurs, it is particularly difficult to identify it in its early stages. We have looked at the factors which can put you at increased risk of osteoporosis. If you think you might be at risk, it is important that you seek advice from your doctor.

Although you might not actually have osteoporosis, there are ways to determine whether you are on your way to developing it, in which case you can take evasive action and try to prevent your bone strength from deteriorating further. If you are a friend or relative of someone who you think may be at serious risk of osteoporosis, try to encourage them to go to their doctor. Offer to accompany them for moral support if you feel it is appropriate.

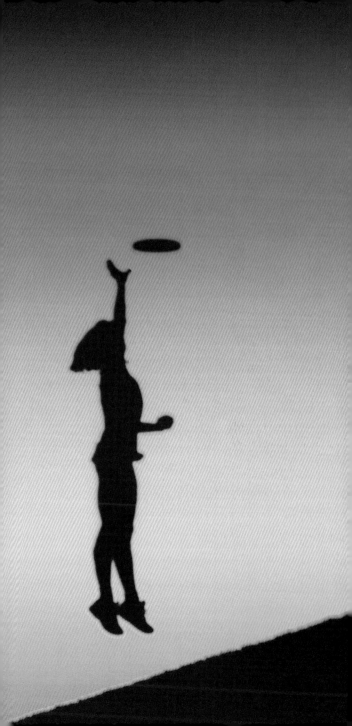

DIAGNOSING OSTEOPOROSIS

If you go to your GP because you suspect that you might have osteoporosis, he or she will ask you what has led you to this suspicion. Your GP will have some background knowledge of your particular medical history, but you might be asked, for example:

- Have your parents or a brother or sister suffered fractures or been diagnosed with osteoporosis?

- Do you find it easy to get about?

- Do you suffer from back pain? Does it come and go?

- Do you have trouble with balance?

- Do you smoke?

- Do you drink much alcohol?

- Did you suffer from an eating disorder when you were younger?

- Have you ever missed periods (apart from when you were pregnant)?

You will be given a physical examination and your doctor may decide to run some blood tests. These can be used to eliminate other possible causes of weak bones, (e.g. cancer or hypogonadism). There are also blood and urine tests available which measure the levels of 'markers' of bone turnover. In other words, these can indicate changes in the rates of bone formation and bone resorption. However, these tests cannot be used to diagnose osteoporosis in the first place, and are usually only used in clinical trials to assess the effectiveness of a new drug.

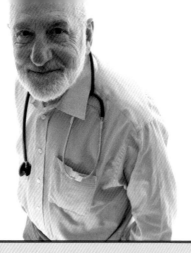

GP

As your GP, I will be responsible for co-ordinating your care in the long-term. You may come and see me because you are concerned that you may have or may be at risk of osteoporosis, in which case I can refer you for diagnostic tests at the hospital. Alternatively, you may have already received emergency medical attention for a fracture, and come to me afterwards for more long-term care.

As well as prescribing medications, I can offer you advice, reassurance and further explanation should you require it. Following your initial diagnostic tests in hospital, I may refer you back to a hospital-based specialist if your osteoporosis is proving particularly difficult to control or is very severe. Some GPs do, however, have a specialist interest in bone problems and may have less need to refer you. I will work with other members of the healthcare team to ensure that regular reviews and check-ups are arranged for you. These are designed to detect and treat any signs of accelerated bone loss and to ensure that you get the best possible care.

My overall aim is to tailor the management process to suit your individual circumstances.

The only definitive way to diagnose osteoporosis is to measure the density of the bones using a DXA scan.

As we saw earlier, this procedure is usually carried out in a hospital, so you may need to be referred to a specialist in order to have the test, although many GPs now have direct access. In most cases, you should not have to wait more than a few weeks for this scan, though it can be delayed for a number of months if the scanning facility is particularly busy.

Although the DXA scan uses radiation to measure your bone density, the dose is very small – much less than is used in a normal chest X-ray. Usually, the scan will look just at your lower spine and hip, which ensures that you are not exposed to any more radiation than is necessary. The scan should take less than half an hour and all you need to do is lie still on a couch. There is no tunnel involved, you do not need to get undressed and you will not feel any discomfort provided you are able to lie fairly flat.

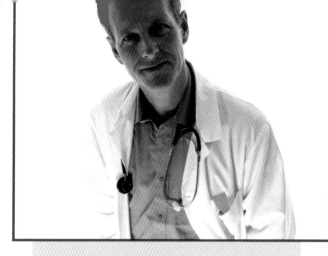

OSTEOPOROSIS SPECIALIST

I am a hospital-based doctor specially trained to manage conditions affecting the bones. If your osteoporosis is proving difficult to control or is particularly serious, your GP may feel that you will benefit from my particular experience in looking after people with osteoporosis and so refer you to me. Also, if your GP suspects that your osteoporosis is secondary to another cause, particularly if you are a man, you might be referred to me for further investigations.

Osteoporosis features in a number of hospital departments, including rheumatology, geriatrics, orthopaedics, endocrinology and gynaecology, and you might encounter me in any number of these. I might also be involved in running special clinics, dealing with fall prevention, for example, along with specialist nurses. Also, if you have any kind of bone-related surgery, a specialist 'orthopaedic surgeon' will be responsible for carrying out the procedure.

Bone density and T-scores

To give it its proper name, the measurement that the DXA scan generates is your bone mineral density. In this form, the measurement is not particularly useful, but the scanner software will use it to calculate a number called your T-score. The T-score basically compares your bone mineral density with the average measurement taken from healthy young adults of your gender. This enables your doctor to determine to what extent your bones have deteriorated. As we have seen, bone strength naturally deteriorates with age, so your T-score is usually negative (that is, your bone mineral density is lower than that of a young adult).

If your T-score is much below zero, though, this will indicate that you are at risk of, or already have, osteoporosis. If you do not yet have osteoporosis, but your bone mineral density is getting low, this is described as osteopenia. If you have osteopenia, this represents an opportunity to make the necessary changes to prevent osteoporosis itself from developing, such as stopping smoking and engaging in regular weight-bearing exercise.

A peripheral DXA (pDXA) scan can measure bone density at the heel or forearm, and so can be used to diagnose osteoporosis. For each scanner, 'normal' limits will have been defined, allowing your doctor to identify whether you:

■ should be reassured that you are fine

■ definitely need treatment

■ will need a further DXA scan – an axial DXA – for a more accurate diagnosis.

pDXA scanners are relatively cheap, portable and easy to use. They can therefore be used in GP surgeries, provided that they are run by a member of staff who has undergone specific training and is registered to use radiation. However, pDXA is only suitable if you are a postmenopausal woman, and it cannot be used to monitor the effectiveness of your treatment.

DIAGNOSIS OF OSTEOPOROSIS BY T-SCORE

Severity	T-score	Fracture risk
Normal	Greater than −1	Low
Osteopenia	Less than −1, but greater than −2.5	Above average
Osteoporosis	Less than −2.5	High

Ultrasound

Ultrasound is a technique in which very high frequency sound waves, unable to be heard by the human ear, are directed into the body. There is no radiation involved in this process. The pattern in which the sound waves are reflected back out again allows an electronic image to be obtained or a measurement to be made. More typically, ultrasound is used to provide images of a baby in the womb, or to scan organs such as the liver or kidneys. However, it can also be used to assess bone structure and strength. Ultrasound is cheaper and more readily available than DXA scanning. Although usually conducted in a hospital, some GP surgeries have access to mobile ultrasound imaging services, so it is possible that you may not need a referral. Ultrasound can be used to give a fairly accurate indication of fracture risk in postmenopausal women and perhaps identify people who should subsequently go on to receive the DXA scan. However, it does not measure bone mineral density and so cannot be used to diagnose osteoporosis or to monitor osteoporosis treatment.

X-rays

Plain X-rays can be used to identify fractures. However, like ultrasound, they cannot be used to provide a definitive diagnosis of osteoporosis as they do not measure bone mineral density. An X-ray may indicate bone thinning, but similar effects can occur simply due to under- or over-exposure of the X-ray film. It is generally claimed that bone density needs to fall by nearly a third before it can reliably be detected on a traditional X-ray.

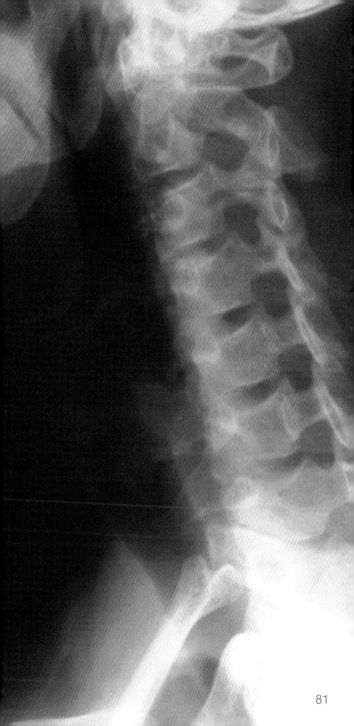

WHAT TO EXPECT

As we have seen, in order to receive a definitive diagnosis of osteoporosis, you will need to be referred by your GP for a DXA scan. The hospital department will send any test results back to your GP and it will be your GP who will work with you to establish an appropriate programme of care. If you do not have osteoporosis but your bones are starting to show signs of weakness (as in the case of osteopenia), your doctor will probably advise you to make some changes to your lifestyle. If your bone mineral density is low enough to give you a diagnosis of osteoporosis, your doctor will combine advice on lifestyle and possibly calcium and vitamin D supplements with a bone-sparing drug treatment. If you have had fractures, you may also need treatment to control your pain. This is also a situation in which your GP may involve a hospital specialist, as you may benefit from their more extensive experience in bone disease.

You need to accept that in the vast majority of cases, osteoporosis does not just 'go away', and whilst there are effective treatments available to slow down the rate at which you are losing bone density, it is unrealistic to expect a complete cure. You will probably need to take calcium and vitamin D supplements and some form of drug treatment for the rest of your life, but this does not mean that you should feel like osteoporosis is controlling your life. Make sure that you are involved in decisions about your treatment – your doctor will be able to take your preferences and circumstances into account when developing a programme of care for you.

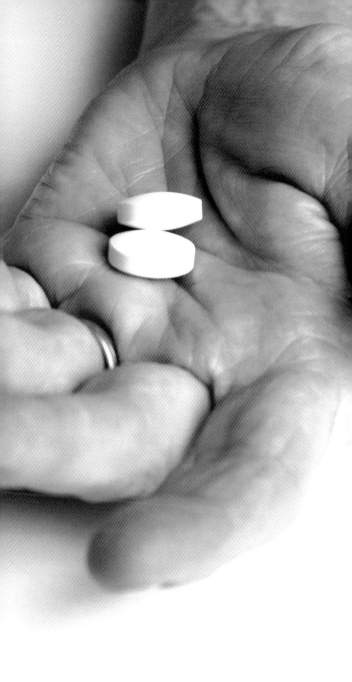

AIMS OF TREATMENT

The various forms of treatment for osteoporosis aim to slow down the rate at which you are losing bone. However, there is a clear relationship between bone density and your risk of fracture. In practice, the outcome that your doctor is aiming for is a reduced rate of fractures, as it is these that affect your quality of life and cause discomfort.

LIFESTYLE CHANGES

As we have seen, your GP will advise you on how you might modify your lifestyle to minimise any further loss of bone density. Even if you have a T-score which is considered to be normal, many of these suggestions would help to prevent you from developing osteoporosis in the future.

Adopt a bone-friendly diet

As everyone knows, it is vitally important to eat a healthy, balanced diet. Guidelines developed for doctors recommend that, of your daily calorie intake:

- 55–60% should be from carbohydrates (found in foods such as cereal, bread, fruit, vegetables and pasta)

- 15–20% should be from proteins (found in foods such as meat, dairy produce and pulses)

- 20–30% should be from fats (found in foods such as oily fish, fatty meat, nuts and cheese).

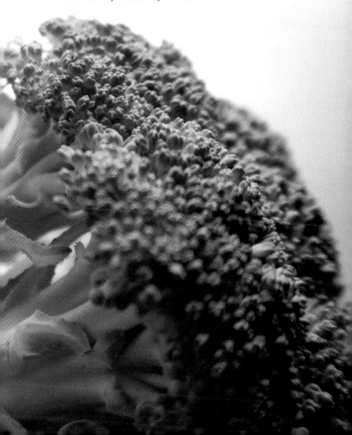

The UK government's Food Standards Agency (*www.food.gov.uk*) has produced a food guide called *The Balance of Good Health*, which shows in what proportions you should aim to eat the five main food groups:

- bread, cereals and potatoes
- fruit and vegetables
- milk and dairy foods
- meat, fish and alternatives
- fatty and sugary foods (fats should mainly be unsaturated, as found in nuts, olive oil, avocados and oily fish, for example, rather than the saturated fats found in foods like fatty meat and cheese).

Maintaining a healthy, balanced diet can be particularly difficult if you have osteoporosis, as your movement may be painful and restricted. If you are struggling to keep up a good diet, speak to a carer or your GP, who will be able to find out about local services that may be able to deliver hot or frozen meals to your door (see *Managing osteoporosis* page 125).

MORE OSTEOPOROSIS MYTHS

It is sometimes claimed that caffeine can increase your risk of osteoporosis and, indeed, there is some evidence that caffeine can cause you to lose more calcium in your urine. However, when caffeine is consumed at normal levels, and with adequate calcium in the diet, there is no evidence for an increased risk of osteoporosis. Caffeinated, fizzy drinks may pose more of a threat than coffee, for example – particularly in childhood if these replace milk intake.

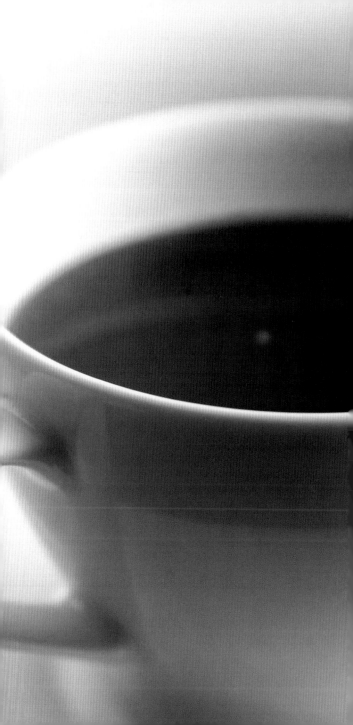

This advice on maintaining a healthy diet is relevant to anyone, regardless of how healthy their bones are. However, if you have osteoporosis, it is particularly important that your diet is providing you with enough calcium and vitamin D.

Calcium

A normal, healthy adult should consume at least 700 mg calcium per day. However, if you have osteoporosis, this recommendation is increased to 1,200 mg. This kind of daily allowance might be difficult to obtain purely by eating plenty of calcium-rich foods, so it may be beneficial to ensure an adequate supply by taking calcium supplements. Your doctor will advise you whether this is appropriate in your particular situation. The values in this table refer to an average daily consumption – it doesn't matter if some days you consume more calcium and some less, as long as over a month or so, your intake averages out at roughly the right amount.

Food	Amount	Calcium content (mg)
Milk	200 mL glass	240
Soya milk*	200 mL glass	26
Fruit yoghurt	125 g pot	170
Milk chocolate	50 g bar	110
White bread	2 x 30 g slices	100
Sardines in oil	60 g	300
Orange	1	70
Boiled spinach	90 g	130
Cheddar cheese	30 g	225

*Most soya milk is fortified to the same level as cow's milk.

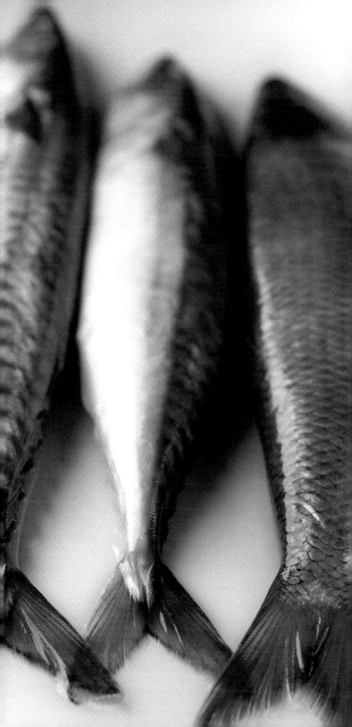

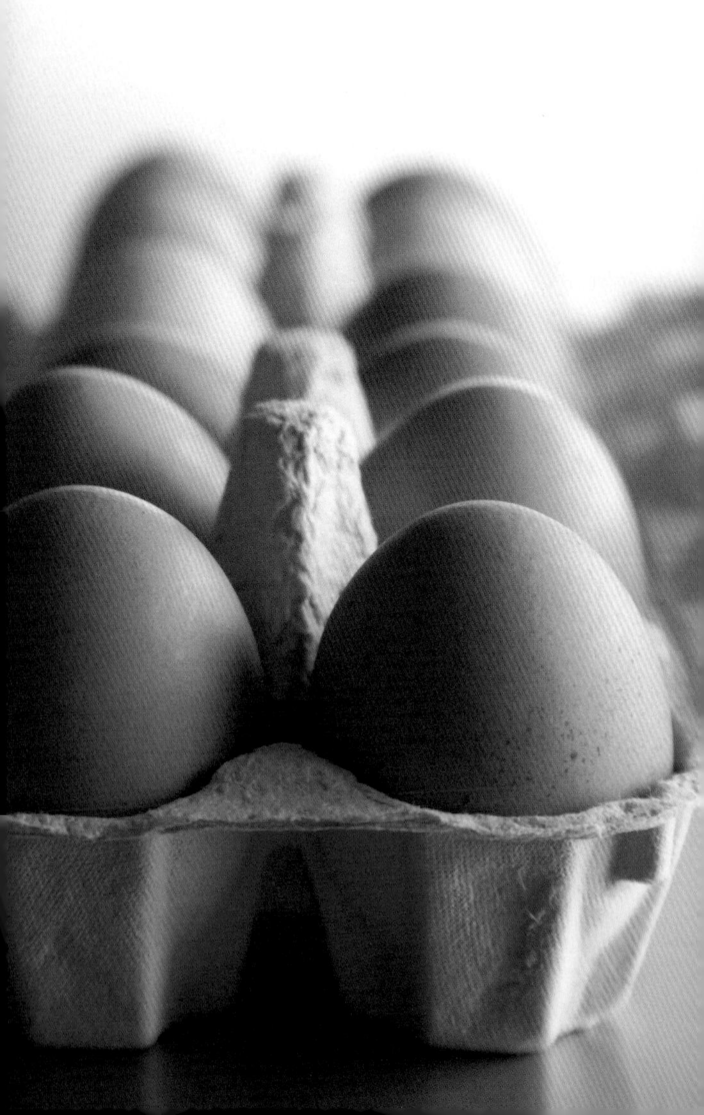

Vitamin D

A typical healthy adult requires about 10 µg of vitamin D per day, whereas 20 µg is the recommended daily intake for a person with osteoporosis. As we have already seen, most of this vitamin D is made in the skin. However, roughly 10% is obtained from your diet. If the skin is receiving very little exposure to sunlight, then it is unlikely that your dietary intake of vitamin D will be enough to compensate for this, and you will probably need to take supplements. It is important to ensure that you are including some good sources of vitamin D in your diet. Some foods, like milk, cereals and margarine are 'fortified' with vitamin D. Foods which are naturally rich in vitamin D include:

- oily fish (mackerel, sardines, salmon, tuna)

- eggs

- liver

- cheese.

As is the case for calcium, there is a limit to the amount of vitamin D that you should ingest. Exceeding the recommended daily amount can be toxic, leading to symptoms such as headache, nausea and constipation.

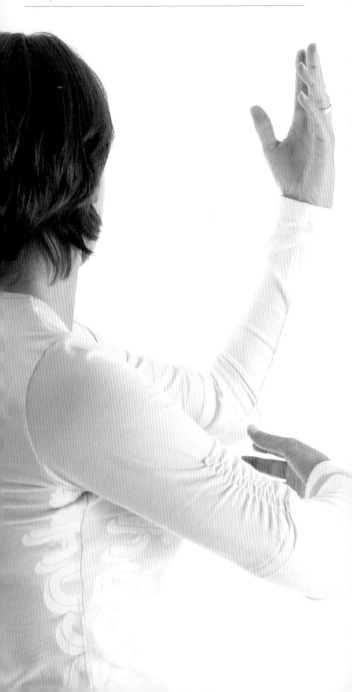

Exercise regularly

It is crucial that children take regular vigorous weight-bearing exercise in order for their bones to develop strength whilst they are growing. Regular activity during childhood and adolescence has been shown to increase the peak bone density achieved in the teens and early twenties. Excessive exercise can be detrimental though, particularly in girls and women. Intensive exercise regimes, particularly if they are associated with poor nutrition, can reduce oestrogen levels, causing periods to start late (delayed menarche) or to stop for a while (amenorrhoea). This greatly increases the risk of bone loss and stress fractures.

Similarly, it is also important for older people to maintain a good level of activity if their bones are to retain their strength. Two types of exercise can be helpful later in life. Vigorous weight-bearing exercise such as aerobics, jogging and skipping can help to improve bone density, and prevent bone loss, as can resistance exercise, such as lifting weights in the gym. For older, frail individuals, balance training and gentle activities such as Tai Chi may improve muscle strength and reduce the risk of falls and fractures. It is important to discuss with your doctor what level of exercise is most appropriate for you – it is important not to put yourself at unnecessary risk of fractures.

Do not smoke

If you smoke, it is really important that you stop. You are probably well aware that smoking increases your risk of heart disease, stroke, lung cancer and many other serious conditions. But did you know that it reduces your oestrogen levels if you are a woman and testosterone levels if you are a man? As we have already seen, low levels of these hormones can lead to osteoporosis. Smoking also has a direct damaging effect on bone-building osteoblast cells.

Cut down on your alcohol intake

Although moderate consumption of alcohol actually appears to be good for bone strength, excessive drinking compromises bone density, probably through effects on the hormones oestrogen and testosterone. Alcohol can also affect the function of vitamin D in your body, thereby disrupting absorption of calcium from your food. Consider, also, the effect that too much alcohol can have on your balance – staggering around in a drunken stupor is hardly a good idea when your bones fracture easily!

	Two units	Three units
Beer (ordinary strength)	1 pint	$1^1/_2$ pints
Wine	2 small glasses	3 small glasses
Spirits	2 single measures	3 single measures
Sherry/fortified wine	2 small glasses	3 small glasses

AIM TO DRINK NO MORE THAN TWO UNITS PER DAY IF YOU ARE A WOMAN AND THREE IF YOU ARE A MAN.

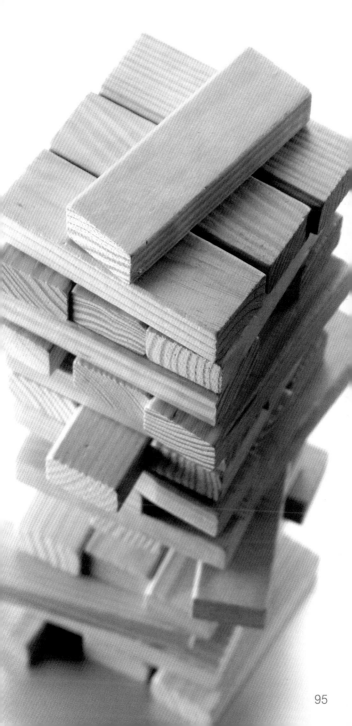

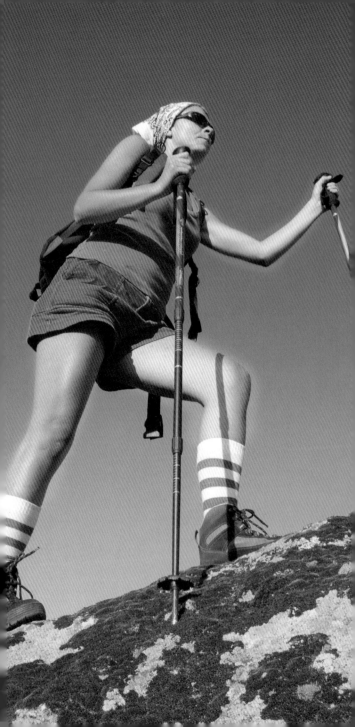

Try to reduce the risk of falls

Aside from avoiding inebriation, there are other measures you can take to try and avoid falls and therefore fractures.

- Minimise clutter on the floors of your home.

- Ensure that rugs are smooth and sealed down so that you don't trip on a corner or edge.

- Fit non-slip mats and grab bars in bathrooms.

- Always turn on lights if you get up during the night.

- Fit non-slip mats in the kitchen and ensure all spillages are mopped up immediately.

- Ensure that there is a secure hand rail next to all stairs.

- Ask your doctor whether any medications you are taking might be affecting your balance, such as those used to treat high blood pressure or heart rate.

- Have your sight tested regularly.

- Wear rubber-soled, low-heeled shoes.

- Use a walking stick if you are unsteady on your feet, particularly when surfaces are uneven.

Your GP will be able to arrange for an occupational therapist to visit you at home and assess whether you need to make changes. If it is agreed that you need to make modifications to your home, your local council should be able to provide practical and, depending on your household income, financial assistance.

DRUG TREATMENTS FOR OSTEOPOROSIS

There are a number of different drug treatments available in the UK for treating osteoporosis. You may need to try more than one of these treatments before you settle on one that suits you. There are various guidelines which a doctor can refer to in order to establish which drugs might be most effective for which patient, including those published by the National Institute for Health and Clinical Excellence (NICE, see *www.nice.org.uk*). Although your doctor will use these guidelines to help him or her make decisions about your care, every individual case is different, and you will need to work together to establish what works best for you. It is likely that you will need treatment for osteoporosis for the rest of your life, so it is important that you get on well with the drug that you have been prescribed.

The drugs and medications referred to in this Simple Guide are believed to be currently in widespread use in the UK. Medical science can evolve rapidly, but to the best of our knowledge, this is a reasonable reflection of clinical practice at the time of going to press.

Source: British National Formulary.

Unless your doctor is convinced that your diet is providing you with adequate calcium and that you are getting enough sunlight exposure to make vitamin D, you will be advised to take calcium and vitamin D supplements.

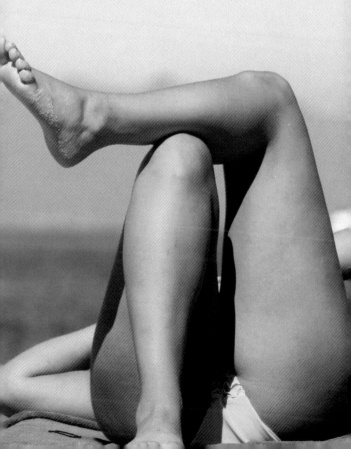

Bisphosphonates

As we saw earlier, bisphosphonates work by reducing the rate of bone resorption. There are four bisphosphonate drugs currently used to treat osteoporosis in the UK:

- alendronic acid (Fosamax®, Fosamax® Once Weekly and Fosavance® [which contains added vitamin D])

- risedronate sodium (Actonel® and Actonel® Once a Week)

- disodium etidronate (Didronel® and Didronel PMO® [which contains added calcium])

- ibandronic acid (Bonviva®).

The most recent NICE guidelines recommend that the first two of these drugs are generally the best options amongst the bisphosphonate drugs, but disodium etidronate may be useful if the first two are unsuitable for any reason or if you experience too many side-effects. The fourth drug, Bonviva®, has only been introduced very recently in the UK, and is not currently covered in the NICE guidelines. This drug offers the advantage that it only needs to be taken once a month, but there is only evidence to show that it protects against vertebral fractures (alendronic acid and risedronate are also proven to protect against hip fractures).

All of these drugs carry specific requirements about how the tablets must be taken, to ensure they are absorbed and to minimise side-effects. They must be taken with a full glass of plain tap water, on an empty stomach, first thing in the morning, and no food, drink or other tablets are to be taken for at least 1 hour. You need to remain upright after taking the tablet to ensure it will pass directly into your stomach and not get stuck in your oesophagus on the way down. The different drugs also vary in the frequency with which you need to take them – ibandronic acid is taken once a month, and alendronic acid and risedronate are now usually given once a week, although daily versions are still available. Your tablets will be accompanied with a patient information leaflet for you to check if you are unsure.

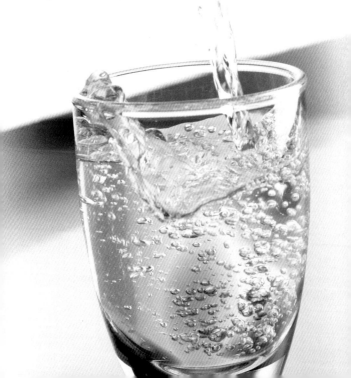

You cannot be treated with bisphosphonate drugs if you have particularly low levels of calcium in your body or if you have certain problems with your kidneys. The most common side-effects associated with these tablets are heartburn and indigestion, but other side-effects include headache, pain in the muscles and joints, constipation, diarrhoea, nausea, abdominal pain and flatulence. Even if you do experience some of these side-effects, they are unlikely to be problematic enough to make you stop taking the treatment. If you are troubled by side-effects, ask your doctor for advice. It is important that you do not simply stop taking your medication without consulting your doctor as there are alternative treatments you can try.

Strontium ranelate

Strontium ranelate, as we have already seen, acts both to reduce the rate of bone resorption and to increase the rate of bone formation. Its brand name is Protelos® and it is supplied as granules which you will need to take in water. Strontium ranelate is not suitable for use by certain groups of people, including those who have serious kidney problems. There are also some other medicines which can interfere with the action of strontium ranelate, so your doctor will take any other medical problems into account before prescribing it. Strontium ranelate does not work as well if it is taken soon after or before food, so it is recommended that it is taken at night, on an empty stomach, avoiding calcium-containing foods and drinks (e.g. milk) for at least 2 hours beforehand.

The most common side-effects of strontium ranelate are headache and diarrhoea, although these usually settle by 3 months into treatment. This drug is also reported to cause eczema or dermatitis in some people. Side-effects are usually mild, though, and tend to go away on their own, given time.

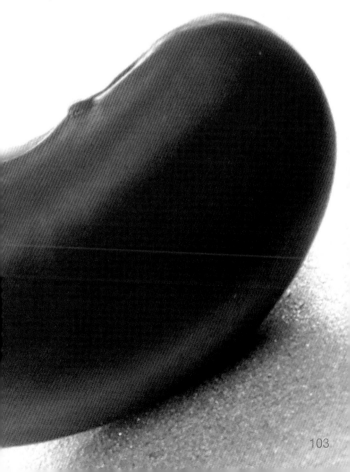

Selective oestrogen receptor modulators (SERMs)

A SERM, as we have already seen, works by mimicking the effects of oestrogen on bone. There is only one such drug currently available for treating osteoporosis in the UK – raloxifene hydrochloride (Evista®) – although there are others in the pipeline. Raloxifene does not appear to be effective in reducing hip fracture rates, but it does prevent vertebral fractures. You will not be prescribed these tablets if you have certain other medical conditions, such as problems with your liver or kidneys. The most common side-effects are hot flushes, leg cramps and flu-like symptoms. As for bisphosphonates and strontium ranelate, side-effects resulting from SERM treatment are not generally serious enough to warrant stopping the treatment, but if you feel that your treatment is causing you problems, you should ask your doctor for more advice. There is a risk that raloxifene hydrochloride can cause blood clots in your veins, so you will not be offered the drug if you have a history of deep vein thrombosis (DVT).

On a positive note, remember that SERMs are labelled 'selective' because they mimic the effects of oestrogen on bone, but reduce the effects of oestrogen elsewhere, such as in breast tissue. Because of this effect at the breast, raloxifene actually appears to reduce the risk of one type of breast cancer in postmenopausal women.

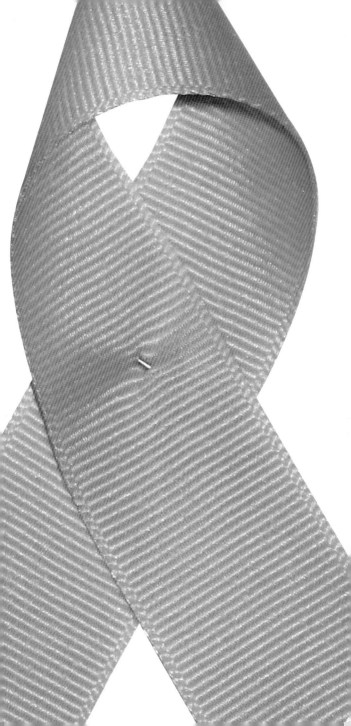

Parathyroid hormone

Parathyroid hormone, in the form of the drug teriparatide (Forsteo®), can be used to treat osteoporosis because, as we have seen, it can increase bone formation if given in small doses on a daily basis. Teriparatide is provided in a pre-filled injection pen and must be injected under the skin. Because of the need for you to learn the injection technique, and the fact that, at present, you can only receive teriparatide for a maximum of 18 months, it is quite unlikely that you will be offered this drug. It is only available for people who have particularly severe osteoporosis and have been unable to tolerate bisphosphonate drugs, or for those in whom these drugs have failed to work. Teriparatide can also cause a number of side-effects, including pain in the limbs, muscle cramps, headache, dizziness, nausea and vomiting, tiredness, depression and vertigo.

Calcitonin

Calcitonin is a hormone produced naturally in the body but a synthetic version (Miacalcic®) is available as a treatment for osteoporosis. The drug, administered by injection or as a nasal spray, promotes the transfer of calcium into the bone. Calcitonin can cause side-effects such as nausea and facial flushing, but importantly can also cause allergic reactions in some people. It is therefore not suitable for anyone with a history of seafood allergies, and is only recommended as a treatment for osteoporosis in non-allergic people when other treatments are unsuitable or have failed to work.

Calcitriol

This drug is an active form of vitamin D and can help in the treatment of osteoporosis. It is available as capsules (Rocaltrol®) and has been used in the past for treating osteoporosis which was caused by taking steroid drugs for other medical conditions. It is, however, rarely used these days.

Hormone replacement therapy

Hormone replacement therapy, or HRT, is used by women around the time of the menopause to relieve symptoms like hot flushes. HRT involves taking tablets or using a skin patch to replenish the hormones oestrogen and progesterone, or just oestrogen if you have had a hysterectomy. It can cause side-effects such as nausea, bloating, weight changes, depression, headaches and cramps, but these are usually tolerable in the short-term. There is also evidence that HRT can cause more serious problems, such as an increased risk of breast cancer, heart disease and stroke. Because of these safety concerns, HRT is no longer recommended for the prevention or treatment of osteoporosis in the UK.

If you are receiving HRT for the treatment of menopausal symptoms, you will benefit from its bone-preserving effects. If other treatments are not proving to be effective or tolerable, your doctor may consider treating your osteoporosis with HRT, but only after considerable discussion with you about the relative risks and benefits of this approach.

TREATMENTS TO HELP CONTROL PAIN

Acute pain

The immediate, acute pain that you might feel when you break a bone can often be relieved a little by:

- resting
- elevating the fractured bone, if in the arm or leg
- applying ice
- keeping the affected bone immobile in a plaster cast
- a nasal spray of calcitonin, which can help with the acute severe pain from a vertebral fracture, though the drug is not licensed for relieving pain.

OFF-LICENCE INDICATIONS

Before they can be used in people, all drugs must be granted a licence by the Medicine and Healthcare products Regulatory Agency (MHRA). The licence will set out exactly which diseases and conditions the drug can legally be used to treat. Any medicinal use of the drug that is not covered in the terms of the licence is called an off-licence indication. Your doctor may prescribe you a drug for an off-licence indication, such as the use of calcitonin for pain relief following an acute vertebral fracture, but this is done at their discretion.

The older style of antidepressants (like amitriptyline [Triptafen®]) are not licensed for pain control in the UK. However, there is strong evidence from clinical trials that some types of these drugs can help to relieve chronic pain by raising the pain threshold by dulling the pain signals being sent to the brain. The doses of antidepressants that are used to relieve chronic pain are much lower than those used to treat people with depression.

Chronic pain

Fractures, particularly those in the spine, can cause more long-term, or chronic pain. If you are suffering from on-going discomfort, your doctor might ask you to rate the severity of the pain on a scale of zero (none) to ten (severe) or may ask you to classify the pain as mild, moderate, severe or excruciating. It may also help to use a visual analogue scale to try and quantify how bad your pain is. These scales are usually 10 cm horizontal or vertical lines with word anchors at each end, such as 'no pain' and 'severe pain'. By marking on the line where you think your pain lies, you are giving your doctor a better idea of its intensity, and repeated scoring of the pain can be used to assess whether treatments are helping. For children, drawings of faces in a series – from smiling (none) to frowning and crying (severe) – can be used to determine the severity of pain.

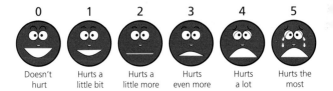

0	1	2	3	4	5
Doesn't hurt	Hurts a little bit	Hurts a little more	Hurts even more	Hurts a lot	Hurts the most

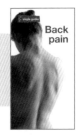

For more information see
Back pain

The options for treating chronic pain are outlined below.

■ **Analgesic drugs** such as aspirin or paracetamol can be effective, but ask your doctor if you think you need to be prescribed something stronger. Analgesics are available as tablets and also as stick-on patches.

■ **Physiotherapy** can teach you exercises that will strengthen your bones and muscles, as well as improving your balance. Exercises done in water (hydrotherapy) can be particularly useful.

■ **Relaxation training or hypnosis** can help to relieve chronic pain.

■ **Transcutaneous electrical nerve stimulation (TENS)** is a technique that cleverly interrupts the 'I hurt' messages that are being sent to your brain from where a fracture has occurred. If these messages, which travel along nerves, do not reach the brain, you do not feel the pain. TENS also stimulates the brain to produce pain-killing hormones called endorphins. The TENS machine is about the size of a personal stereo, and can be clipped to clothing in a similar manner. It has electrode pads which you need to stick to the skin, and although you might feel some tingling whilst the machine is working, this should not be painful or unpleasant. TENS does not work for everyone, and it should not be used at all in some cases, such as if you have a heart pacemaker, or are in the early stages of pregnancy.

If you wish to try TENS, and your doctor agrees that it is suitable for you, you might be able to try a machine for free. If you find it effective, you will need to purchase your own, but make sure you buy one from a reputable source and get proper instructions on how to use it.

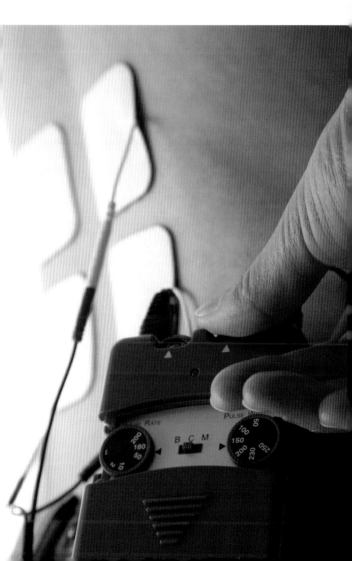

COMPLEMENTARY THERAPIES FOR OSTEOPOROSIS

Osteoporosis lends itself to a number of complementary therapies. These treatment options, as suggested by their name, are designed to complement the more conventional treatments, not to replace them. Many complementary therapies have not been subjected to the same rigorous tests for effectiveness and safety as the drug treatments, and so it is wise to be cautious about whether a particular treatment is worthwhile and safe for you, given your symptoms and your medical history. If you are considering trying one, talk to your doctor to find out if it is suitable for you and whether they can refer you to an NHS practitioner or recommend a reputable private one.

- **Acupuncture** is an ancient Chinese practice that is growing steadily in popularity in the UK. By inserting fine needles into your 'channels of energy', the practitioner aims to improve your overall well-being. There is evidence that acupuncture offers particular benefits in pain relief, and the technique is becoming increasingly available on the NHS.

- **Reiki** is a Japanese word meaning 'universal life energy'. A Reiki treatment involves the practitioner transferring this energy to areas of the body which they feel to be lacking in it, through touch. This is believed to stimulate the body's own healing processes. However, there are claims that the technique can work over distance too, without the need for direct touch.

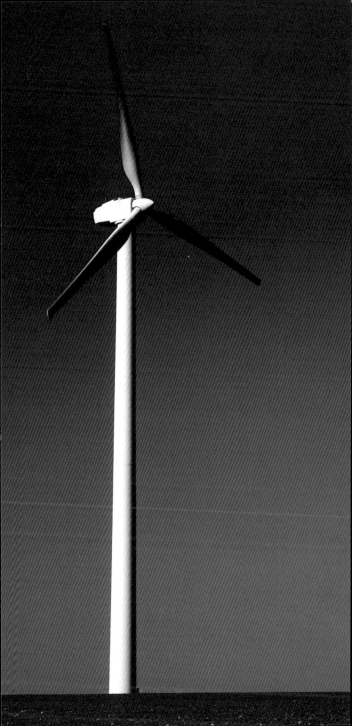

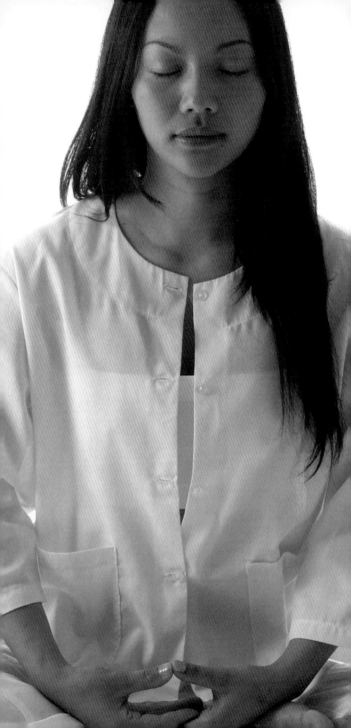

■ **Homeopathy** is based on the concept that 'like cures like'. An agent which causes relevant symptoms in a healthy individual is then given to a patient in a hugely diluted form. The treatments used are so weak that you could argue that they would be completely ineffective. A homeopathist, however, believes that it is the vibrational energy of the treatment, rather than the actual chemical content, which causes the effects.

■ **Aromatherapy** is a technique in which essential (very concentrated) plant oils are applied to the skin, often by massage, but also sometimes as bath oils. Less commonly, the oils are inhaled. It is thought that the smell of the oils may have a relaxing effect in the brain, and oils crossing the skin may act at the cause of the problem – in this case, the bones.

■ **Reflexology** involves applying manual pressure to regions of the foot, and less often the hands. It is based on the belief that all parts of the body are said to be reflected in the feet and hands. Reflexologists claim that crystalline deposits of waste products from the rest of the body collect in the foot. By working on a particular point where crystals have collected, the therapist aims to heal the corresponding area of the body.

Treatment of secondary osteoporosis

As we have already seen, osteoporosis is described as secondary when it occurs as a complication of another medical condition or its treatment. Many of the conventional drug treatments for osteoporosis are suitable for treating these cases, but sometimes it may be possible to reduce the rate of bone loss by treating the underlying condition or changing the medications being used. It may be possible, for example, to take breaks in steroid treatment, and perhaps change the way that the drug is taken, such as using creams or inhalers instead of tablets. Problems with the gastrointestinal system and eating disorders such as anorexia nervosa and bulimia can reduce the amount of calcium reaching the bones. Overcoming these problems using the relevant drug treatments or counselling programmes, and perhaps taking calcium supplements, will help to keep the bones strong in these cases. Similarly, hypercalciuria is a condition in which too much calcium is lost in the urine. This disorder must be treated in order that the bones receive enough calcium.

There are many other ways in which treating a medical condition or changing the drugs you are taking can indirectly improve bone strength in secondary osteoporosis. Your doctor will explore all of the possible ways of improving your condition, but it is important that you help him or her by being honest about the possible factors that may have contributed to the condition, such as eating disorders or alcohol misuse.

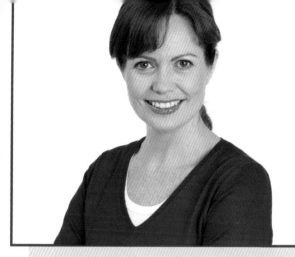

SPECIALIST NURSE

As a nurse who specialises in bone problems, I have a number of possible roles in the management of your osteoporosis. Traditionally, I am based in the hospital, where I provide support for doctors who specialise in osteoporosis and carry out certain practical aspects of your treatment. I am responsible for the practicalities of the DXA scan, ensuring that you are in the correct position and comfortable for your scan.

I may also have a major role in running osteoporosis clinics, which provide you with the opportunity to ask questions about the practicalities of your care – how best to avoid fractures, how to obtain help in the home and suchlike. I will generally have time available to discuss with you the lifestyle changes that might help you to manage your osteoporosis.

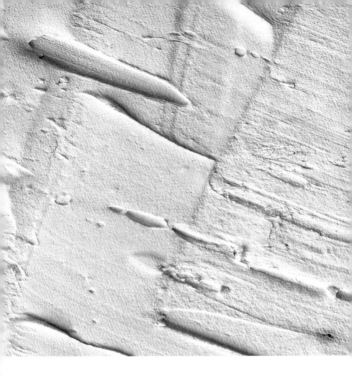

TREATMENT OF FRACTURES

Bones are pretty good at healing themselves, but if you do suffer a fracture, the healing process can be helped a little. The way that the fracture is managed will depend on where the fracture has occurred. If a bone in your arm or leg is broken, a doctor or nurse at the hospital will be able to immobilise it with a plaster cast, to ensure that the bone stays in the correct position while it is healing, and that you do not put too much pressure on it before it is strong enough to cope.

If you suffer a hip fracture, you will usually need surgery to restore your mobility. This might involve the insertion of metal pins, or even a total hip replacement (usually comprising a combination

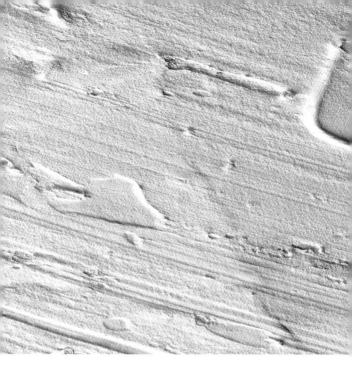

of plastic cement and stainless steel). You will probably not be able to put your full weight on your hip for at least 10 weeks after the operation.

If you have a vertebral fracture, your doctor may advise that you undergo a procedure called vertebroplasty. You will lie on your front while the vertebroplasty is carried out. It involves injecting your broken vertebra with a kind of plastic cement, through a long needle, to restore the bone structure. You will have a scan before, and probably after the procedure, in order to check where the cement needs to be positioned. Vertebroplasty is normally done in the morning, and takes less than two hours. You should be able to leave the hospital on the same day, and will only need about 24 hours of bed rest.

Very similar to vertebroplasty is another promising treatment for vertebral fractures called kyphoplasty. This also involves injecting plastic cement into the fractured bone to restore its structure, but during kyphoplasty, little balloons are inserted into the bone and inflated until they fill the space created when the bone fractured. When they are the right size and shape, they are filled with the plastic cement, which hardens and restores the bone structure as in vertebroplasty. Both of these procedures can improve the shape of the spine, reduce the risk of future fractures, and importantly, provide effective pain relief.

BONE HEALING

Bone is quite unique within the body because, after it has been damaged, such as in the case of a fracture, it repairs itself by creating replacement bone. This is unlike the skin or muscles, for example, which form scar tissue when they are damaged, rather than replacing like with like.

In the first few days after a fracture, the affected area will be sore and swollen, as your body strives to get rid of damaged tissue and fragments of bone. Following that, the repair process occurs over a period of weeks or months, adding bone which is initially soft and rubbery, and later becomes harder as it gains calcium. This new bone is called the callus, and initially forms a lump around the affected area, as a kind of temporary repair. However, for a number of months after the repair is complete, the bone is remodelled to refine its shape. The callus is replaced by stronger bone and the bone eventually looks like it did before the fracture occurred.

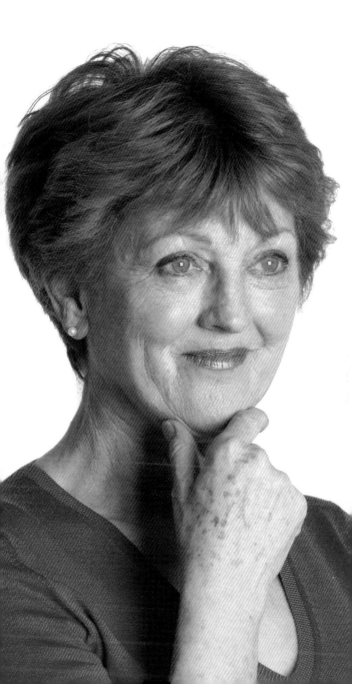

MANAGING OSTEOPOROSIS IN CHILDREN

As osteoporosis is so rare in young people, there is not a lot of experience in how best to treat it. Certain drugs, such as the bisphosphonates, are thought to offer some benefit, but use of these drugs in children is off-licence, and must be overseen by a specialist. The focus is on maintaining a diet rich in calcium and vitamin D and doing plenty of weight-bearing exercise. In most cases, osteoporosis in children has a known cause, such as an eating disorder or steroid treatment for another condition, such as asthma. In some cases, it will be possible to treat the underlying condition, or change the medication that is to blame, thus improving osteoporosis indirectly. Most children who suffer from idiopathic juvenile osteoporosis tend to improve over time anyway, although their adult height may be affected as osteoporosis during childhood can affect a child's growth.

MANAGING OSTEOPOROSIS IN MEN

As we have already seen, osteoporosis can occur in men as well as women, albeit less commonly. If you are a man with osteoporosis, it is likely that it is secondary to another health problem or its treatment. Because of this, your doctor may spend some time investigating possible underlying causes, and perhaps ask for specialist help in doing so. The lifestyle and dietary advice that is given to women with osteoporosis also applies to men, but there is much less experience of treating osteoporosis in men with drugs, so a specialist is likely to be involved in deciding which treatments are suitable.

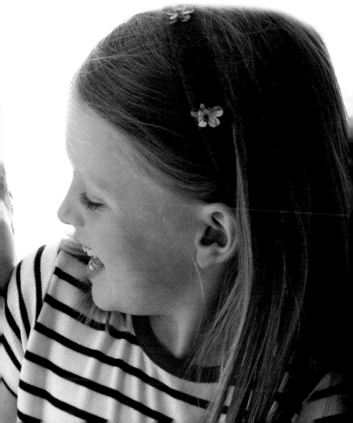

MANAGING OSTEOPOROSIS IN PREGNANCY

The drugs available for treating osteoporosis are not generally recommended to be used by pregnant women or those who are breast-feeding, because there is not enough evidence to prove that they are safe for the baby. Osteoporosis associated with pregnancy usually improves on its own once breast-feeding is complete, and so management of the condition during this time is usually focused on maintaining a bone-friendly diet together with calcium and vitamin D supplements.

BENEFITS AND SERVICES

You and your carers might be entitled to certain benefits and services which will help you with the day-to-day costs and difficulties of living with osteoporosis. There are various organisations that may be able to help you to find out whether you are entitled to help. The contact details of the Benefits Enquiry Line is listed at the end of this book (see *Simple extras* page 134). In addition to medical care services, such as home-based rehabilitation from a physiotherapist, you may be entitled to practical help, in the form of home-delivered meals, for example, although these services are unlikely to be offered free of charge.

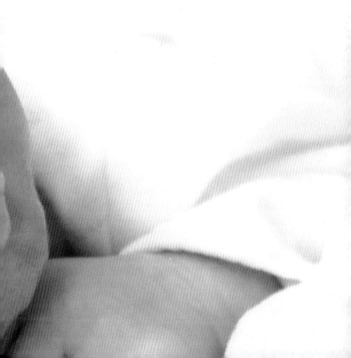

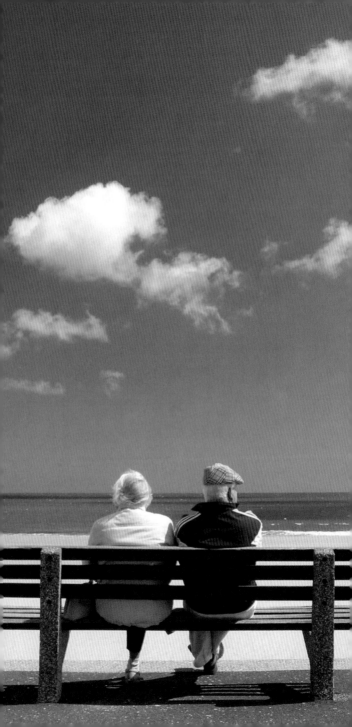

SUPPORT FOR CARERS

If you have osteoporosis, and particularly if you are elderly, it is likely that you are cared for not only by medically trained healthcare professionals but also by a relative or friend or by another volunteer carer. The day-to-day support that a carer offers can be invaluable, helping out with tasks requiring mobility that you no longer have and providing general emotional support. It is important that your carer is cared for too! Although they choose to look after you, and clearly want what is best for you, it requires a lot of time and dedication on their part, and they are bound to have other commitments of their own. If they are a close relative or friend, they will probably find it emotionally draining too, as they don't want to see you suffer.

The National Osteoporosis Society (*www.nos.org.uk*) co-ordinates an extensive network of over 130 Regional Support Groups across the UK. These offer support and help to raise funds both for sufferers of osteoporosis and, importantly, their families and carers. Getting involved with one of these groups will not only benefit you and your carers, but is also likely to help existing members of the group, as you can share your experiences with them and offer your own support.

THE LONG AND SHORT OF IT

Is it serious?

Unfortunately, osteoporosis can be a serious condition. Complications occurring after fractures can, in the worst cases, cause death, and the fractures themselves can be painful and debilitating. Even if you are not experiencing painful symptoms and are not bothered by your osteoporosis at the moment, it is vital that you appreciate how serious it might become in the future, and the importance of sticking to your programme of care.

What should I expect?

There are a range of different treatments available for minimising any further deterioration of your bones. The important thing is to spot osteoporosis as early as possible, so if you are at all concerned, it is best to speak to your doctor. You are unlikely to know about it until you suffer a fracture, and even this might go unnoticed. By taking medications as directed by your doctor, and ensuring that you eat a healthy diet and take enough appropriate exercise, you should be able to keep your osteoporosis under control. Make sure you take an active role in managing your condition, and maintain as much independence as you can. Your friends and family will be able to support you, both practically and emotionally. However, it might be worth enquiring about a volunteer carer if you need more help than your friends and family can reasonably offer you.

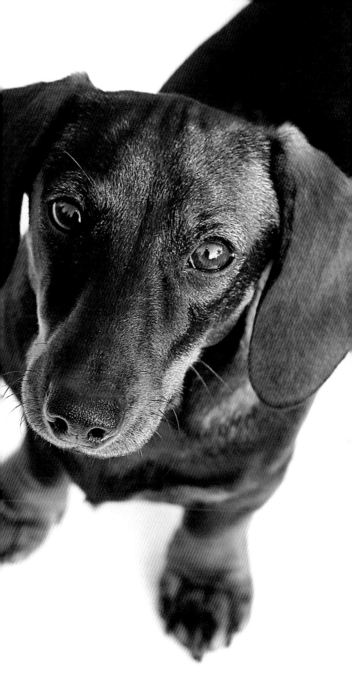

GETTING THE MOST OUT OF YOUR HEALTH SERVICE

Osteoporosis is a long-term condition and it is important that you work together with your doctor to optimise your care. Maintaining a good relationship with your GP, specialist or any other healthcare member you may come into contact with, is fundamental to managing your osteoporosis effectively. These people will be able to explain to you why you are in pain, teach you how best to manage your pain and help to relieve your pain by physical manipulation or drug treatment. It is important that you remain in regular contact with your GP, and keep them informed of any improvement or deterioration in your symptoms. Remember, if one management approach fails to work, there are many others that can be tried.

- Don't be afraid to ask for help or advice.

- Keep your doctor informed of all the treatments you are taking, including dietary supplements.

- Know what to expect and when to ask for help.

- Consider bringing a carer along to your doctor's appointments so that they can be kept up to speed on any changes to your care programme.

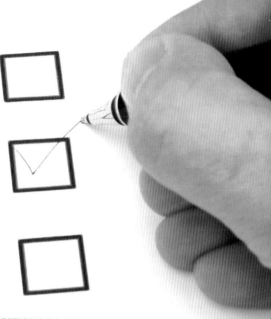

QUESTIONS TO ASK YOUR DOCTOR

Having a doctor's appointment or going to the hospital for tests can be quite a daunting prospect. It is often helpful to write down a list of questions before you attend your appointment.

■ How serious is my osteoporosis?

■ Might I have had fractures in the past without realising?

■ What signs should I look out for to identify fractures in the future?

■ What precautions should I take to avoid falls at home?

■ Should I make changes to my diet?

■ What sort of exercise should I be doing?

■ How often should I come back for appointments?

■ How can I find out about getting extra help at home?

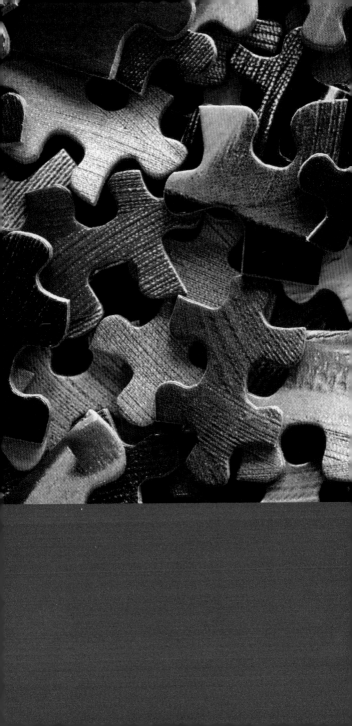

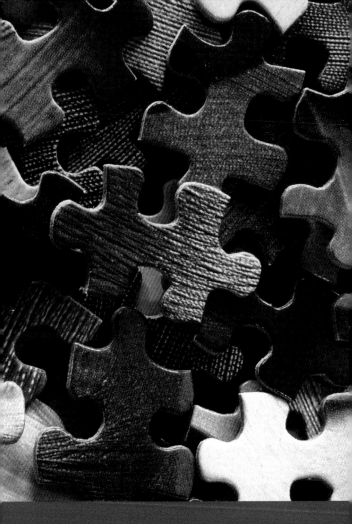

Simple extras

FURTHER READING

■ **BESTMEDICINE Osteoporosis**
CSF Medical Communications Ltd, 2005
ISBN: 1-905064-81-0, £12.95
www.bestmedicine.com

■ **Back pain (Simple Guide)**
CSF Medical Communications Ltd, 2005
ISBN: 1-905466-01-3, £5.99
www.bestmedicine.com

■ **Arthritis (Simple Guide)**
CSF Medical Communications Ltd, 2006
ISBN: 1-905466-12-9, £5.99
www.bestmedicine.com

■ **Thyroid disorders (Simple Guide)**
CSF Medical Communications Ltd, 2006
ISBN: 1-905466-09-9, £5.99
www.bestmedicine.com

USEFUL CONTACTS

■ **Benefits Enquiry Line (BEL)**
Tel: 0800 882200
Textphone: 0800 243355
Website: *www.dwp.gov.uk*

■ **British Acupuncture Council (BAcC)**
63 Jeddo Road
London W12 9HQ
Tel: 020 8735 0400
Email: *info@acupuncture.org.uk*
Website: *www.acupuncture.org.uk*

The British Reflexology Association
Monks Orchard
Whitbourne
Worcester WR6 5RB
Tel: 01886 821 207
Email: *bra@britreflex.co.uk*
Website: *www.britreflex.co.uk*

Carers UK
Ruth Pitter House
20/25 Glasshouse Yard
London EC1A 4JP
Tel: 0808 808 7777
Email: *info@carersuk.org*
Website: *www.carersuk.org*

The Disabled Driver's Association
Ashwellthorpe
Norwich NR16 1EX
Tel: 0870 770 3333
Email: *hq@dda.org.uk*
Website: *www.dda.org.uk*

Disabled Living Foundation
380/384 Harrow Road
London W9 2HU
Tel: 0845 130 9177
Email: *info@dlf.org.uk*
Website: *www.dlf.org.uk*

Disability Rights Commission (DRC)
FREEPOST MID02164
Stratford upon Avon CV37 9BR
Tel: 08457 622633
Textphone: 08457 622644
Website: *www.drc-gb.org*

■ **National Osteoporosis Society**
Camerton
Bath BA2 0PJ
Helpline: 0845 4500230
General enquiries: 01761 471771
Email: *nurses@nos.org.uk*
Website: *www.nos.org.uk*

■ **NHS Direct**
NHS Direct Line: 0845 46 47
Website: *www.nhsdirect.nhs.uk*

■ **The Patients Association**
The Patients Association is a UK charity which represents
patient rights, influences health policy and campaigns
for better patient care.
Contact details:
PO Box 935
Harrow
Middlesex
HA1 3YJ
Helpline: 0845 6084455
Email: *mailbox@patients-association.com*
Website: *www.patients-association.com*

SIMPLE GUIDE QUESTIONNAIRE

Dear reader,

We would love to know what you thought of this Simple Guide. Please take a few moments to fill out this short questionnaire and return it to us at the FREEPOST address below.

CSF Medical Communications Ltd
FREEPOST NAT5703
Witney
OX29 8BR

SO WHAT DID YOU THINK?

Which Simple Guide have you just read?

_____

Where did you buy it (store/town)?

_____

Who did you buy it for?

☐ Myself   ☐ Friend   ☐ Relative
☐ Patient   ☐ Other

Where did you hear about the Simple Guides?

☐ They were recommended to me   ☐ Internet
☐ Stumbled across them   ☐ Other

Did it meet with your expectations?

☐ Exceeded   ☐ Met all
☐ Met most   ☐ Fell below

Was there anything you particularly liked?

_____

_____

_____

Was there anything we could have improved?

_____

_____

_____

WHO ARE YOU?

Name: _____

Address: _____

_____

_____

Tel: _____

Email: _____

How old are you?

☐ Under 25   ☐ 25–34   ☐ 35–44
☐ 45–54   ☐ 55–64   ☐ 65+

Are you...   ☐ Male   ☐ Female

Do you suffer from a long-term medical condition? If so, please specify.

_____

WHAT NEXT?

What other topics would you like to see covered in future Simple Guides?

Thanks,
    the Simple Guides team